Baillière's
CLINICAL
PAEDIATRICS

INTERNATIONAL PRACTICE AND RESEARCH

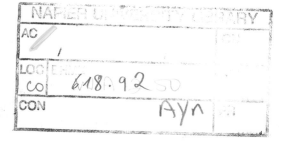

Baillière's

CLINICAL

PAEDIATRICS

INTERNATIONAL PRACTICE AND RESEARCH

Volume 5/Number 3
August 1997

Unintentional Injury in Childhood and Adolescence

A. AYNSLEY-GREEN MA, DPhil, MBBS, FRCP(Lond), FRCP(Edin), PRCPCH
S. N. JARVIS MD, FRCPH
I. ROBERTS MBChB, MRCP, PhD
E. M. L. TOWNER MA, BSc, PhD
Guest Editors

Baillière Tindall
London Philadelphia Sydney Tokyo Toronto

This book is printed on acid-free paper.

Baillière Tindall
W.B. Saunders
Company Ltd

24–28 Oval Road
London NW1 7DX, UK

The Curtis Center, Independence Square West,
Philadelphia, PA 19106–3399, USA

55 Horner Avenue
Toronto, Ontario M8Z 4X6, Canada

Harcourt Brace & Company
Australia
30–52 Smidmore Street, Marrickville, NSW 2204, Australia

Harcourt Brace & Company
Japan Inc
Ichibancho Central Building,
22–1 Ichibancho, Chiyoda-ku, Tokyo 102, Japan

Whilst great care has been taken to maintain the accuracy of the information contained in this issue, the authors, editor, owners and publishers cannot accept any responsibility for any loss or damage arising from actions or decisions based on information contained in this publication; ultimate responsibility for the treatment of patients and interpretation of published material lies with the medical practitioner. The opinions expressed are those of the authors and the inclusion in this publication of material relating to a particular product, method or technique does not amount to an endorsement of its value or quality, or of the claims made by its manufacturer.

ISSN 0963–6714

ISBN 0–7020–2319–1 (single copy)

Baillière's Clinical Paediatrics is published four times each year by Baillière Tindall.
Prices for Volume 5 (1997) are:

TERRITORY	ANNUAL SUBSCRIPTION	SINGLE ISSUE
Europe including UK	£95.00 (Institutional) post free	£30.00 post free
	£52.00 (Individual) post free	
All other countries	Consult your local Harcourt Brace & Company office	

The editor of this publication is Gail Greensmith, Baillière Tindall,
24–28 Oval Road, London NW1 7DX, UK.

Baillière's Clinical Paediatrics is covered in Index Medicus, Current Contents/Clinical Medicine, Current Contents/Life Sciences, the Science Citation Index, SciSearch, Research Alert and Excerpta Medica.

Baillière's Clinical Paediatrics was published from 1972 to 1986 as *Clinics in Paediatrics*

Typeset by Phoenix Photosetting, Chatham.
Printed and bound in Great Britain by the University Printing House, Cambridge, UK.

Contributors to this issue

A. AYNSLEY-GREEN MA, DPhil, MBBS, FRCP(Lond), FRCP(Edin), FRCPCH, Nuffield Professor of Child Health, Institute of Child Health, University College London Medical School, 30 Guilford Street, London WC1N 1EH, UK.

J. A. EYRE BSc, MBChB, DPhil, FRCP, FRCPH, Professor of Paediatric Neuroscience, The Department of Child Health, The Sir James Spence Institute of Child Health, The Royal Victoria Infirmary, Queen Victoria Road, Newcastle upon Tyne NE1 4LP, UK.

ROB FORSYTH PhD, MRCP, DCH, Senior Lecturer in Paediatric Neurology, Department of Child Health, University of Newcastle upon Tyne, Royal Victoria Infirmary, Newcastle upon Tyne NE1 4LP, UK.

MICHAEL HAYES BSc, PhD, Projects Director, Child Accident Prevention Trust, Clerk's Court, 18–20 Farringdon Lane, London EC1R 3AU, UK.

STEPHEN N. JARVIS MD, FFPHM, FRCPCH, Professor of Community Child Health, Department of Child Health, Institute of Child Health, University of Newcastle upon Tyne, UK.

J. C. LAWRENCE PhD, CBiol, FIBiol, Senior Research Fellow, Wound Healing Research Unit, University of Wales College of Medicine, Llandough Hospital, Penlan Road, Llandough, South Glamorgan CF64 2XX, UK.

SARA LEVENE MS, MB BChir, MRCP, MRCPCH, Medical Consultant, Child Accident Prevention Trust, Clerk's Court, 18–20 Farringdon Lane, London EC1R 3AU, UK.

JONATHON P. NICHOLL BA, MSc, CStat, HonMFPHM, Director, Medical Care Research Unit, University of Sheffield, Regent Court, 30 Regent Street, Sheffield S1 4DA, UK.

JIM NIXON BSocWk, MSocWk, BA, PhD, Senior Lecturer in Medical Social Work, Department of Child Health, University of Queensland, Royal Children's Hospital, Herston, Queensland 4029, Australia.

JOANNE OZANNE-SMITH MBBS, MA(Prelim), MPH, FAFPHM, Senior Research Fellow, Accident Research Centre, Monash University (MUARC), Victoria, Australia.

BARBARA M. PHILLIPS FRCP, FFAEM, Consultant in Paediatric Emergency Medicine, Accident and Emergency Department, Alder Hey Children's Hospital, Eaton Road, Liverpool L12 2AP, UK.

I. BARRY PLESS CM, MD, FRCP(C), Professor, Departments of Pediatrics and Epidemiology & Biostatistics, McGill University, The Montreal Children's Hospital, 2300 Tupper Street, Room C-538, Montreal, Quebec H3H 1P3, Canada.

KEITH M. PORTER FRCS, DipIMC, RCS(Ed), Consultant Trauma and Orthopaedic Surgeon, Selly Oak Hospital, Raddlebarn Road, Birmingham B29 6JD, UK.

CAROLYN A. REID MBBS, FRCS(C), Consultant Plastic Surgeon, Royal Victoria Infirmary & Associated Hospitals NHS Trust, Queen Victoria Road, Newcastle upon Tyne NE1 4LP, UK.

Editorial Note

The presentation of material in *Baillière's Clinical Paediatrics* has been updated, and we hope that the changes will make the information in the series more accessible to readers.

Each chapter is now preceded by a short abstract summarizing the content and by keywords that will be used for indexing and abstracting purposes.

Where the author has identified the most important references cited in the chapter, these have been indicated in the reference list with asterisks.

IAN ROBERTS MBChB, MRCP, PhD, Senior Lecturer in Epidemiology and Director, Child Health Monitoring Unit, Institute of Child Health, 30 Guilford Street, London WC1N 1EH, UK.

PETER W. ROWE MBBS, Senior Registrar in Paediatric Neurology, The Department of Child Health, The Sir James Spence Institute of Child Health, The Royal Victoria Infirmary, Queen Victoria Road, Newcastle upon Tyne NE1 4LP, UK.

JO R. SIBERT MA, MB BChir, DCH, DObst, RCOG, MD, FRCP, FRCPCH, Professor of Community Child Health, Department of Child Health, University of Wales College of Medicine, 1st Floor, Academic Centre, Llandough Hospital, Cardiff, South Glamorgan CF64 2XX, UK.

ELIZABETH M. L. TOWNER MA, BSc, PhD, Senior Lecturer in Community Child Health, Community Child Health, University of Newcastle upon Tyne, Donald Court House, 13 Walker Terrace, Gateshead NE8 1EB, UK.

JANETTE K. TURNER BSc, RN, Research Fellow, Medical Care Research Unit, University of Sheffield, Regent Court, 30 Regent Street, Sheffield S1 4DA, UK.

SEAN WALSH MRCPI, MSc, DCH, Consultant in Accident and Emergency Medicine, Leeds General Infirmary, Great George Street, Leeds LS1 3EX, UK.

HEATHER WARD BSc, MSc, Principal Research Fellow, Centre for Transport Studies, University College London, Gower Street, London, WC1E 6BT, UK.

DAVID W. YATES MD, MCh, FRCS, FFAEM, Professor of Emergency Medicine, University of Manchester and Honorary Consultant, Hope Hospital, Department of Accident and Emergency Medicine, University of Manchester, Hope Hospital, Salford M67 8HD, UK.

Table of contents

PREVIOUS ISSUES

FORTHCOMING ISSUE

Preface

Unintentional injury is the single greatest threat to life for children and adolescents after infancy in the UK (Table 1). The matter must be of primary interest to our whole society. This issue reviews, for Paediatricians, selected aspects of injury prevention, the management of acute injury, and the longer term consequences of injury in childhood.

The Introductory chapter sets the broader national scene, highlighting the paucity of academic and professional interest in the subject within the UK. This should cause great concern to our policy makers and to health

Table 1. Deaths in childhood and adolescence from unintentional injury (ICD E800–E949)* in England and Wales in 1994.

	0–4 years		5–9 years		10–14 years		15–19 years	
	M	F	M	F	M	F	M	F
Total (E800–E949)	107	74	85	31	106	49	376	124
Motor vehicle traffic accidents (E810–E819)	20	25	54	22	64	40	274	96
Involving collision with pedestrian (E814)†	11	16	31	12	35	22	26	22
Pedal cyclist involved in collision with MV (E813.6)†	0	1	9	1	11	5	14	2
Other transport accidents (E800–807: 820–848)	2	2	4	0	9	1	9	2
Fire and flames (E890–899)	16	13	5	2	1	3	2	1
Drownings and submersion (E910)	21	6	5	2	1	0	14	1
Accidental falls (E880–888)	5	4	4	0	5	1	16	1
Accidental mechanical suffocation (E913)	5	2	3	0	15	0	7	1
Inhalation and ingestion (E911 & 912)	15	11	3	2	2	0	3	2
Poisoning (E850–869)	4	2	0	1	0	1	38	17

* ICD Codes E800–849 are used in this table. Injuries caused by violence and self-harm are excluded. This definition is used in *The Health of the Nation: Key Area Handbook on Accidents* (Department of Health, 1993)
† Both included in motor vehicle traffic accidents.
Source OPCS: 1994 Mortality Statistics, Series DH2 No: 21: England and Wales (HMSO, 1996).

professionals alike. Later chapters reveal that in other countries some of these problems have been surmounted, where they have managed to place injury prevention and control high on their health policy agendas.

One characteristic of these successful countries has been the importance they attach to data collection and its use in evaluation—the subject of the first chapter. There is a clear requirement that the evidence for successful injury prevention and control is founded on accurate data. Both at the level of the descriptive information for monitoring and local planning and to allow for more formal evaluations of preventive intervention, current data systems are weak. On the other hand, the evaluation techniques are relatively well developed and their use is illustrated in this and in subsequent chapters across a variety of injury prevention settings (home, leisure and road).

Chapter 2 outlines the evidence concerning the prevention of child injuries in the home setting. This is a crucial issue for pre-school children and the few evaluated and effective interventions are described in some detail, with the focus on the most severe and/or frequent injuries.

Those injuries which are more common amongst an older group of children are discussed in Chapter 3. The evidence concerning the burden and preventability of injuries in playgrounds, during various sports/leisure activities, by drowning, and while in formal occupations at school and work is reviewed.

Chapter 4 looks in more detail at the single most significant setting for severe and fatal injuries amongst children of all ages—road traffic. The subtle interactions between child development, gender, behaviour variations, supervision, and the hazards presented by the actors, vehicles and the built features of the road environment are dissected. The evidence for effective intervention is reviewed, in particular the requirement for a mix of legislative, educational and environmental approaches.

The literature cited in these early chapters highlights the imbalance between countries in their attention to this dominant problem of injury in childhood—both at the academic and public service investment levels. Chapter 5 looks in more detail at how this situation has arisen and the lessons we can learn from those practitioners and policy makers who have already acted successfully to prevent injury.

Despite the best of preventive efforts, childhood injury will remain a major health issue, and the second half of the book addresses the important issues of treatment and rehabilitation. Chapter 6 highlights the importance of a structured approach to the management of the injured child, in both the pre-hospital and the hospital phases, whereas Chapter 7 addresses how the organization and delivery of trauma services can contribute to improving outcome. Specifically, Chapter 7 considers whether the model of the 'Trauma Centre' that has been developed most fully in the USA, is applicable to paediatric populations in other countries.

Most child injury deaths are from head injuries and Chapter 8 reports an audit of the management of children after fatal head injury. Chapter 9 takes up a similar theme asking why have injury death rates fallen over the past decades.

Children under 15 comprise 45% of burn and scald admissions, with those under 2 years being the highest risk group. The effective management of thermal injury in childhood has the potential to avoid a substantial burden of disfigurement and disability. In Chapter 10 the practical management of the paediatric burn is outlined, with particular emphasis on first aid, resuscitation, dressing and wound care.

Finally, Chapter 11 addresses the critically important issues surrounding the rehabilitation and support for head injured children and their families. There can be little doubt that rehabilitation after head injury is a major but neglected aspect of the child injury problem. Although the provision of an effective and seamless rehabilitation service for brain injured children must be regarded as a priority for health services, this final chapter gives an insight into just how far we will have to go to achieve this.

We hope that this issue will help to highlight the importance of the issue of unintentional injury in childhood and stimulate practitioners, policy makers, and researchers in their efforts to decrease the tragic morbidity and mortality to children from injury.

'If a disease were killing our children in the proportion that accidents are, people would be outraged and demand that this killer be stopped.' (Dr C. Everett Koop, US Surgeon General).

A. AYNSLEY-GREEN
S. N. JARVIS
I. ROBERTS
E. M. L. TOWNER

REFERENCE

The National Safe Kids Campaign (1989) *Safe Kids are No Accident Leader Guide*. Washington, DC: Safe Kids.

Introduction

Unintentional injury in childhood and adolescence—an introductory perspective

A. AYNSLEY-GREEN MA, DPhil, MBBS, FRCP(Lond), FRCP(Edin), FRCPCH

Nuffield Professor of Child Health
Institute of Child Health, University College London Medical School, 30 Guilford Street, London WC1N 1EH, UK

Unintentional injury in childhood and adolescence is one of the most important problems affecting the health of children in our contemporary society. Its consequences should be of immense concern to any national Government involved in the planning and delivery of effective healthcare services for this age group. In the UK, the recent Report by the House of Commons Health Committee on the State of the Health of the Nation's Children has firmly emphasized the significance of injury and the need for further research into its causation as well as into aspects of prevention and the management of injured children (HCHC, 1996–1997). This current focus is to be welcomed greatly, but it is fair to say that until recently the full significance of the consequences, ranging from the national economic burden caused by injuries to the effects on individual children have not had a high priority either in Government policy or in the league table of desirable topics for research (DoHCD, 1991).

It is a pleasure, therefore, to be one of the editors of this issue, the purpose of which is to provide an opportunity for leading experts world-wide to give their personal perspective of aspects of this major health issue. It is hoped that the issue will become a reference source for those interested in learning more of the subject, as well as providing provocative comment for those already engaged in its prosecution.

The title of this introduction uses the phrase *unintentional injury* rather than the more common use of the word *accident*. It could be argued that one of the reasons why there has been so little focus on this aspect of child health is that the word *accident* itself implies an inevitability, an event which is outside the control of individuals, and which is such a common event as to naturally demand the provision of health care resources. There is an immediate need to educate not only the general public but also those engaged in public health policy so that it is recognized that many injuries to children are preventable. Moreover, even when they occur, increased focus on the training of those involved in the management of children may

Baillière's Clinical Paediatrics —
Vol. 5, No. 3, August 1997
ISBN 0–7020–2319–1
0963–6714/97/030325 + 4 $12.00/00

improve substantially the outcome for those injured children (Sharples et al, 1990).

The hard statistics concerning the occurrence of child injury are shocking. Thus, child injury deaths in the age group 0–19 years within England and Wales were responsible for 1422 deaths in 1992, accounting for nearly half of all deaths in this age group with a steep inverse social class gradient (DiGuiseppi and Roberts, 1997). Whilst there has been a most welcome reduction in the rate of injury deaths in children aged 0–15 years between 1981 and 1991, it is immensely disappointing to see how this fall is not reflected in the most disadvantaged social classes in our society (Roberts and Power, 1996). These facts are identified in Table 1.

Table 1. Injury death rates/100 000 children (age 0–15 years).

Social class	Rate		% Decline
	1981	1991	
I	24.2	16.5	32
II	25.0	15.8	37
III (non-manual)	24.2	19.1	21
III (manual)	35.7	34.3	4
IV	47.5	37.8	21
V	84.7	82.9	2

P value for trend, $P < 0.001$.

In addition to injuries being the leading cause for deaths in children and adolescents, they are also the cause of substantial hospital morbidity and long-term permanent disability (Barker et al, 1996).

Table 2 outlines the numbers and percentages of children aged 5–14 years with hospital morbidity and from both Tables 1 and 2 it could be calculated that the economic cost to the Health Service in dealing with both the costs of children who die and those who have ongoing morbidity is massive. Whilst most children with injuries recover, nonetheless, it has been estimated that 3.2% of injuries requiring hospital treatment in young

Table 2. Hospital morbidity (HES, England 1993–1994).

5–14 years	N	%
Respiratory diseases	83 749	17.5
Injury and poisoning	76 586	16.0
Nervous system/sense organs	62 922	13.2
Digestive system diseases	61 198	12.8
Ill defined conditions	42 656	8.9
Genitourinary diseases	27 318	5.7
Congenital anomalies	23 824	5.0
Neoplasm	19 368	4.1
Musculoskeletal diseases	19 023	4.0
Mental disorders	14 170	2.9
Diseases of the blood	11 663	2.4
Infectious and parasitic diseases	11 604	2.4
Skin diseases	10 640	2.2
Endocrine	9498	2.0

people over the age of 16, cause permanent disability, while 9.7% of patients admitted to hospital with injury experience permanent disability as a result of that injury.

These bald facts reinforce strongly the view that injury really is a major health issue and that there is urgency in addressing the causes and consequences of such events. There is an undisputed need for research. However, what is the capacity of the research community at present to respond to the challenge of performing research in this vital area?

The report of the Special Advisory Group set up by the Department of Health in 1994 to advise on NHS Priorities for Mother and Child Health identified injury as one of the key fields for research effort (CRDC, 1994). Over £6 million was provided by the Department of Health to commission research in the national priority fields, and invitations to bid for this money were invited from the research community. The response was gratifying in the sense that of all of the commissioned programmes to date by the Department of Health, this proved by far to be the most popular with well over two thousand enquiries being received culminating in outline submissions from over 694 research groups (MCH, 1997).

An analysis of the numbers of applications submitted for each of the research fields revealed a depressing picture with reference to unintentional injury in childhood and adolescence. Thus, whilst the largest number of applications related to aspects of high technology medicine, especially in the intensive care of sick newborn infants, the topic of injury received the lowest number of applications. At the end of the commissioning process only four projects relating to injury were funded.

Thus, despite being the most important cause of death and handicap in children outside the newborn period, and despite the enormous economic and social cost, the UK at present has a research community in child health which has major problems in asking relevant questions and delivering credible research.

As the Chairman of the Advisory Group responsible for the Report on Priorities for the NHS in Mother and Child Health, it is a special pleasure to join with three other colleagues who are acknowledged experts internationally in the field to edit this issue of *Baillière's Clinical Paediatrics*.

As mentioned above, I join with colleagues in hoping that the issue will not only focus on the scale of the problem of unintentional injury in childhood and adolescence, but stimulate heads of Academic Departments of Paediatrics and Child Health to encourage young researchers to develop interests and skills in this most important facet of contemporary child health.

A. AYNSLEY-GREEN

REFERENCES

Barker M, Power C & Roberts I (1996) Injuries and the risk of disability in teenagers and young adults. *Archives of Diseases in Childhood* **75:** 156–158.

CRDC Advisory Group (1994) *Improving the Health of Mothers and Children NHS Priorities for Research and Development*. London: Department of Health.

(DoHCD) Department of Health Consultative Document (1991) *The Health of the Nation*. London: HMSO.

DiGuiseppi C & Roberts I (1997) Injury mortality among children and teenagers in England and Wales, 1992. *Injury Prevention* **3:** 47–49.

(HCHC) House of Commons Health Committee (1996–1997) *The Specific Health Needs of Children and Young People. Session 1996–97*. Vol. 1. Second Report. London: HMSO.

(MCH) Mother and Child Health (1997) *R & D Newsletter for the National Programme on Mother and Child Health*. Issue 1.

Roberts I & Power C (1996) Does the decline in child injury death rates vary by social class? *British Medical Journal* **313:** 784–786.

Sharples PM, Aynsley-Green A, Storey A & Eyre JA (1990) Avoidable factors contributing to the death of children from head injury. *British Medical Journal* **300:** 87–91.

1

Data and evaluation

STEPHEN N. JARVIS MD, FFPHM, FRCPCH

Professor of Community Child Health
Department of Child Health, Institute of Child Health, University of Newcastle upon Tyne, UK

JOANNE OZANNE-SMITH MBBS, MA(Prelim), MPH, FAFPHM

Senior Research Fellow
Accident Research Centre, Monash University (MUARC), Victoria, Australia

Useful data result in action to prevent or better manage injuries. Evaluation demonstrates the effects of such action. The range of routine data sources that may be analysed to specify causes and consequences of childhood injury is described. Issues of data quality and desirable enhancements to those datasets are examined. Paediatricians have a crucial and largely unrealized rôle in the generation and use of these data. Examples are given of the application of established evaluation techniques in a variety of child injury settings. Most injury prevention and control measures in childhood still await such elucidation.

Key words: mortality; morbidity; epidemiology; evaluation

Data and evaluation are interdependent. Evaluation requires an intervention and a method to estimate attributable changes. Injury data should so describe circumstances and consequences that interventions may be specified and their effects demonstrated. In short, data are virtually useless without a link to action. Action may be useless unless evaluated with data. For convenience, we will split the subject but the essential link is there.

DATA: INTRODUCTION

This section asks a number of questions that we hope will turn the dry business of injury data collection into the exciting challenge that it can become. These data are important, are available, should be complete and accurate, and need careful analysis. Paediatricians will find themselves to be vital partners in their collection, interpretation and use.

Baillière's Clinical Paediatrics—
Vol. 5, No. 3, August 1997
ISBN 0–7020–2319–1
0963–6714/97/030329 + 17 $12.00/00

Why are data important?

The over-riding purpose of injury data is to achieve and to demonstrate actual prevention of injury (or its consequences). By understanding the relative frequency and circumstances of injury we can specify and target appropriate preventive interventions. Accurate measurement of injury frequency and severity may demonstrate that these interventions have an effect. With an account of the original case-mix and ultimate outcomes of those children who continue to suffer injuries, the effects of various patterns of management will be decipherable. On all these counts, our current injury data systems, particularly those in the UK, are weak.

What data are available?

'—to help decide what measures to take to prevent child head injury.' This rider is added as data have no meaning without a practical focus. The answer can be managed by considering those data that provide evidence concerning both the burden of this injury and its preventability.

Head injury is frequent and occasionally very severe. These are the two components of the 'burden' and the sources of relevant data are numerous. Head injury is one of the commonest causes of *hospital admission* in childhood (DoH, 1996a); it accounts for a large part of the huge resources consumed by children attending *emergency rooms* [accident and emergency departments] (Walsh et al, 1996); it is the principal reason for emergency *intensive care* (Sharples et al, 1990b) of children: and it is the largest single reason for *fatal* (OPCS, 1993) injury in childhood.

The preventability of these injuries makes greater demands on the data. Head injuries are largely attributable to falls during domestic or leisure activities (*Consumer Product Surveillance*) (DTI, 1994) or to collisions in or with motor vehicles (*road traffic accident (RTA) records*) (DoT, 1994; Sharples et al, 1990b). There are many clues in these routine data sources concerning potentially avoidable causes of head injury (e.g. babywalkers, excessive vehicle speed etc). To penetrate further, a detailed review of *Coroners' records* (Levene, 1991) may be required, together with an assessment of the avoidable factors from *clinical records* (Sharples et al, 1990a). Systematic and critical appraisals of the *literature* (Dowswell et al, 1994) concerning the effects of preventive intervention may substantiate the degree to which this massive injury burden can currently be prevented. Fundamental research will be required to identify preventive measures for the residual injuries.

These data sources cited above are not accessible with equal facility in different countries (and England and Wales systems will be referred to principally). Their common characteristic is that they can inform *local and national* policy and practice. This is largely because, where they are available, they attempt to cover 100% of the incident injuries of this type. The sources can be categorized as health, vital statistics, road traffic or national surveillance systems (often sample based).

Medical attendance or '*health*' records concerning children with injuries may be completed by personnel from ambulance [emergency service], primary care, accident and emergency (A&E) [emergency room, ER] departments, inpatient or specialized units (Intensive Therapy; burns etc). The crucial questions are: can these data be retrieved electronically? Are they complete for residents of an area? What detail is reliably collected about key variables such as age, sex, diagnosis (International Classification of Disease (ICD) 'N' ± severity), mechanism of injury (ICD 'E'), date, time and place of event, and the home address postcode [Zip code] of the victim (Jarvis et al, 1996). In the UK these health data are only commonly available for inpatients through Hospital Episode Statistics (DoH, 1996a,b). They are sometimes recorded in *Trauma Registries* for those in intensive care (Yates et al, 1992) and are occasionally accessible through computerized A&E systems. However these latter two sources are frequently institution rather than population based.

With respect to *vital statistics* (mortality and population data) the picture is much better. Virtually 100% of deaths are ICD 'E' coded, individual level material is available and a number of local and national level statistical reports from the Office for National Statistics and other agencies are produced (OPCS, 1995a,b). These include decennial supplements (OPCS, 1988) where census based denominators and aggregated death data are combined. Census based counts (OPCS, 1991) of the population by age, sex and key social characteristics are also readily obtained down to Enumeration District [Census tract] level to allow calculations of rates of injury by person, place and time.

The last comprehensive and long running source of child injury event data is that collected by the police and local road traffic authorities concerning *road traffic accidents* (DoT, 1994). Despite the lack of home postcode and ICD level diagnostic coding, this source contains some of the most detailed injury circumstance data of any source. There are regular local and national level analyses, some of which make use of travel survey and vehicle registration data as alternative rate denominators (e.g. injuries/100 000 vehicle km).

National level sample data concerning injury in childhood are also collected routinely in many countries. The two principal models of this type are product safety surveillance systems (DTI, 1994) and population health surveys which include questions concerning injury (e.g. in the General Household Survey: Breeze et al, 1991). In the UK, additional relevant surveys (sample or policy level) are also conducted concerning injury seen in primary care (Royal College of General Practitioners & OPCS, 1995), during fires (Home Office, 1992) and at work (HSE, 1995).

What other data sources could be useful?

Risk factor data

A carefully documented case series of injured children attending hospital

(MUARC, 1993) may reveal patterns of associated factors or injury circumstances that point to an obvious form of preventive intervention. The importance of such data cannot be overstated, especially when they cover large populations and are used to follow trends over time.

However, the interpretation of the risk factor data collected in this way can occasionally be misleading. For instance, boys in England attend hospital twice as often as girls with cycling injuries, cycling fatality rates are four times higher in Holland than in the UK, and amongst young men in England and Wales fatal head injuries while cycling are commoner than while horse riding. In each statement, the lack of data concerning exposure to known risks amongst the source population for cases creates a false impression. First, the exposure specific risk of cycling (injuries/unit time spent cycling) is really the same for boys and girls (Towner et al, 1994). Second, cycling is actually more than twice as dangerous/km in England than in Holland (Mynors and Savell, 1992). Third, horse riding mortality is nearly 20 times greater/unit of participation in horse riding than while cycling (Avery et al, 1990: i.e. the relative risk is greater). Furthermore, injury prevention campaigns such as cycle helmet legislation can achieve overall reductions in injury frequency by reductions in exposure (e.g. cycling) as well as a specific reduction in head injury frequency due to lowering of the risk while actually cycling (Vulcan et al, 1992).

The collection of such relevant exposure prevalence data in the source population by direct observation is expensive although very informative. More cost effective sampling techniques have been developed recently for observational studies of road traffic exposure of pedestrians and cyclists (Drummond and Ozanne-Smith, 1991). Methods have also been developed to obtain this material using self-completion questionnaires to describe generic risk prevalence amongst school aged children (Towner et al, 1994). In some circumstances, data collected for other purposes can provide population level exposure data to help interpret injury event material (e.g. travel surveys (DiGuiseppi et al, 1997; DoT, 1994), sports insurance policies (Kujala et al, 1995), consumer product sales (Kraus, 1985)).

Economic data

Demonstrating that injuries can be reduced in frequency or severity as a result of intervention, although desirable, is insufficient. For competitive resource allocation decisions, the cost of the intervention and the avoided costs* or values† of the preventable injuries are also needed.

Few data are available except in the road safety field concerning intervention costs: for instance there are no routine data concerning the cost of Public Health programmes intended to prevent injury. Some progress has

---

* Health Sector costs plus indirect costs such as lost work productivity to parents, property damage, legal costs etc.
† Valuation of life or persistent disability may add a considerable extra amount beyond 'avoided costs' onto the benefit side from successful interventions.

been made to obtain values for an avoided death or non-fatal injury, particularly in the road safety field (Jones-Lee, 1993). These have been used extensively to justify investment in road safety engineering/vehicle design and other interventions using cost/benefit models. It should be noted here that even in the more restricted analyses where the cost of intervention is set against the avoided costs of injury there can be very substantial 'profits' from investment in prevention (J. Mackenzie, 1996).

Increasing effort is also being directed to achieving a cost model for the huge financial burden and potential outcomes from prevention and management of other forms of injury (e.g. consumer product safety investments).

Severity of injury

Surveys to ask people about injuries in the previous 2 weeks must address the issue of minimum severity: 'Do you mean this graze?' Ascertainment of *all* incident injuries in a population using A&E or Inpatient data can only be achieved by setting a minimum level of severity and ignoring a group of cases with relatively minor injuries who may or may not attend or be admitted to hospital (Walsh et al, 1996). Determining the effect of a preventive intervention (e.g. cycle helmets) that attenuate the degree of injury without altering the frequency of impacts will require a measure of injury frequency at different levels of severity. Comparing different forms of treatment for injury depends on allowance for the original case-mix. Accounting for the economic burden of particular causes of injury (e.g. consumer products) will be very sensitive to the distribution of severity of the resulting injuries as well as to their absolute frequency.

For all these reasons it is highly desirable that injury data systems include a simple measure of severity of the original injury (i.e. not dependent on treatments such as length of stay). The best established general method is the Abbreviated Injury Scale (AIS: American Association for Automotive Medicine, 1985) from which is derived the Injury Severity Score (Baker et al, 1976). Other methods may be required for very minor, for very severe, and for some special types of injuries (e.g. suffocations and drowning). AIS can be mapped with reasonable reliability from (ICD 9 CM) diagnostic codes (MacKenzie et al, 1986) but otherwise requires specific coding to be undertaken. Considerable development work is under way to improve injury severity measurements as predictors of death and impairment (E. MacKenzie, 1996).

What are the important issues in data quality?

Injury data can be incomplete, or inaccurate, or both. 'Completeness' may involve the original ascertainment of the injury incident (an issue fundamentally related to case definitions and severity—see above) or can refer to the absence of some items amongst the circumstantial data (Walsh et al, 1996).

'Inaccuracy' has various components, but operates generally to reduce validity. Retrospective accounts of injury can be very inaccurate after a few weeks (Peterson et al, 1993) Coding of type, cause and severity of injury can vary with coders' experience, with the coding system used, and with the quality of the original clinical records (Langley, 1982; MacKenzie, 1984). Assignment of social status etc by reference *via* postcodes to the average characteristics of the area in which people live can introduce errors (including ecological fallacy) (Morgenstern, 1982; Reading and Openshaw, 1993).

Making the connections between the recording clinician, the coding process and the uses of the data (both for clinical audit and wider preventive epidemiology) is a major contributor to accuracy. Adding narrative text to computerized records will also allow more flexible analysis while improving face validity.

How can injury data be analysed?

First check for completeness and consider some of the possible sources of inaccuracy. It is usually appropriate to analyse injury data disaggregated by age group and sex—age in particular has a profound effect on the places and circumstances in which childhood injuries are likely to occur. The nature and broad causes of injury may be separated out to focus attention on appropriate prevention measures (e.g. head injuries while cycling). The analysis can proceed by considering the influence of other recorded risk factors relating to person (social group, behaviour, height), place (home/school, area of residence), activity (working, playing sport, in-line skating) and time (of day, year). Important information concerning preventable causes may also come from a careful account of the avoidable circumstances surrounding the injury event itself (for instance using Haddon's Matrix: Haddon, 1973).

For most analyses it is essential to relate the injury event sub-groups to their denominator (source population) in the form of a rate (e.g. comparison of the annual rates of cycling head injury/10 000 boys aged 5–9 as between one city and another). To emphasize the true importance of the child injury burden in a population a useful alternative is to express frequency as a rate of potential life years lost.

In the absence of denominator data, case series data may be useful to determine relative frequencies (proportions) of particular types of injuries, although potential biases must be identified.

Further refinements to analysis become possible when injury event records from different sources are linked (e.g. road traffic accident data and hospital data), when service resources are also accounted for (e.g. length of stay, investigations) and when long runs of data can compare trends in injury over time with parallel changes in protective or causal factors.

What are the implications for clinicians?

Paediatricians have a long history of attention to the social and environmental origins of poor health in childhood. With some exceptions, this has not extended to unintentional injury, at least not at a scale commensurate with the cause of 50% or more of all child deaths in developed countries.

The first implication for paediatricians is that recognition of the true importance of injury will justify a serious interest in the data necessary to examine this huge problem.

Paediatricians are already in command of many of the best data available concerning injury in childhood. However, those in a strong position to influence the most important causes of these injuries are often not from the health sector. It is vital that injury prevention is based on the best information concerning injury frequency and circumstances. The second implication is therefore that paediatricians work with local and national injury prevention organizations to ensure their data is used and useful.

Last, there is a way in which paediatricians can act directly on the basis of the data. There is no more powerful and respected children's advocate in the community. Let data put informed passion into your call for action on behalf of children.

EVALUATION: INTRODUCTION

With the availability of injury data of sufficient quality to identify major problems and the concurrent identification of potentially effective interventions, it is timely to examine the rationale and methods for the evaluation of interventions to prevent injury. The various levels of evidence of effectiveness from process to outcome evaluation, and the contribution each can make will be examined. While many public health interventions produce health outcomes only after many years, injury prevention measures, such as design changes and regulation, can be expected to result in lower injury rates in targeted populations in the relatively short term.

The quality of evidence is dependent on the methods used, including the use of experimental or statistical controls, demonstrating statistical significance (indicating that the effect is unlikely to have occurred by chance) and minimizing bias in the design. Each major method for injury prevention evaluation is briefly outlined and illustrated with an example from the injury prevention literature.

While the concepts of evaluation are relatively simple, decisions about the choice of method, potential biases and research design issues, including sample size, and statistical significance are complex. It is strongly advised that researchers and implementers involve epidemiological and/or statistical advice on evaluation from the outset in any research design.

Ideally, evaluations are undertaken by independent researchers, who are not responsible for the intervention.

Why evaluate?

Evaluation provides scientific evidence of the effectiveness of an intervention. Since there are usually two components to an intervention, a counter-measure and an implementation process, it is necessary to address both, to the extent possible. In some cases, the effectiveness of the counter-measure will already have been determined and the evidence published. Biomechanical, as well as epidemiological, evidence of the effectiveness of counter-measures and the absence of associated unwanted effects is highly desirable, where appropriate.

Evaluation is necessary in order to determine whether an intervention is effective in reducing injury rates or severity; or reducing risk factors; whether an intervention should be implemented more widely; for the purposes of accountability to funders; and to prioritize interventions in terms of relative effectiveness. It may also identify unanticipated or unwanted effects of the intervention (Robertson, 1980). In addition, evaluations provide the basis for cost/benefit analyses on which policy decisions may be made.

What is evaluation?

Evaluation of injury interventions addresses clearly articulated research questions, encompassing the aims and objectives of the intervention in order to measure and describe the achievements (lack of achievements) of the intervention. These should relate to impact and outcomes wherever possible, and secondarily to processes. It is not sufficient to know that a particular population or portion of that population has been exposed to an intervention. Nor is it sufficient to know that a reduction in injury rate occurred. It is necessary to know that exposure to a counter-measure or implementation programme actually leads to injury prevention (has a causal association) or reduction in risk factors (impact) and, for the purposes of replication and cost/benefit analyses, to know how the outcome was achieved.

The necessary components of the evaluation of a public health inter-vention are generally:

- Structure (context assessment)
- Process
- Impact or intermediate and surrogate
- Outcome
- Documentation

What is structure evaluation or context assessment?

This phase of evaluation is a combination of a needs analysis and assess-ment of the infrastructure and other resources available to an intervention, also referred to as 'community diagnosis' (Schelp, 1988). It is conducted before the intervention and constitutes an evaluation for project design (Sherrard, 1995). First it defines the injury problem and assesses its importance and the feasibility of intervention. It also assists with identify-ing target groups, determining implementation processes and provides baseline data against which to measure change. In addition to informing the implementation process, this part of the evaluation contributes to the development of guidelines for replication.

What is process evaluation?

Process evaluation determines how impacts and outcomes are achieved or explanations for failure to achieve them. Sherrard (1995) describes process evaluation as relating to the strategies of the interventions programme or programme delivery.

Feedback from process evaluation on issues such as reach, or penetration, of the programme, throughout the intervention period, provides the opportunity to review and enhance strategies.

What is impact or intermediate evaluation?

Impact evaluation determines whether or not programme objectives relating to risk factor reductions are achieved. The reasons for using such intermediate measures, where prior evidence of a strong relationship exists between the intermediate measure and the desired outcome, are several. Injuries, particularly those resulting in death, are relatively rare events in a particular population. Hence, intermediate measures are required to monitor the effectiveness of interventions. This can be a powerful form of evaluation if the counter-measure implementation or hazard reduction, which is measured as the intermediate step in reducing injury, has been proven to be effective in reducing injuries in independent studies. Examples of such counter-measures include swimming pool fences, smoke detectors, playground equipment of fall height less than 1.5 m, and baby-walkers designed not to fall down stairs.

Changes in behaviour, attitudes and knowledge may be a weaker measure, since a two-stage intermediate process may be required to actually prevent injuries.

What is surrogate evaluation?

Surrogate criteria for injury outcome evaluations are a substitute group of injuries which may be a sub-set or super-set of the specific desired outcome (if that is unavailable) and/or evidence exists of a strong relationship between the two (Cameron, 1995).

What is outcome evaluation?

Outcome evaluation relates to the injury reduction aims and objectives of an intervention. It generally measures changes in the rate or severity of injuries. Where injuries are frequent and the counter-measures and implementation methods are successful, injury reductions can be expected in the relatively short term and can be demonstrated by well designed evaluation studies (Walton, 1982 Guyer et al, 1989).

Both the impact and outcome evaluations can contribute to cost/ benefit analyses to determine the financial return on the investment of resources over the period of study. This information can be useful in supporting funding proposals for continuing or expanding the programme, or in comparing this intervention with other intervention programmes.

Why is documentation essential?

Documentation of all aspects of the intervention including aims, objectives strategies and implementation allows interpretation of the evaluation results, comparison with other interventions and transfer of the methods. It may also allow the study to contribute to a meta-analysis.

What contribution can the physical sciences make?

Evaluation methods of the physical sciences, such as biomechanics, physics, chemistry and engineering, may contribute particularly to the evaluation of counter-measures. They generally involve measurement of a physical property under a range of conditions and provide proof in the form of physical measurement and replicability.

Biomechanics, for example, provides scientific evidence of force attenuation and can be used to optimize counter-measure design by determining which designs are most effective (e.g. shin guards for soccer, hockey and other relevant sports), or to determine what properties are required to withstand the forces of objects and particles with particular physical characteristics and velocities (e.g. for the design of eye protection).

What is the difference between formative and summative evaluation?

While summative evaluation simply reports on the effectiveness of an intervention, formative evaluation plays a more interactive role in the intervention process. Formative evaluation also makes recommendations for future studies.

What evaluation methods are available?

There are several major methods for evaluation applicable to injury prevention, and others will need to be developed to deal with new requirements as the discipline progresses. For example, with regard to community-based injury prevention and other health promotion programmes, institutionalization is an important objective for programmes and components of programmes that are proven to be effective. Quantified and validated instruments are required to measure its effectiveness.

The challenge for the researcher is to choose an appropriate evaluation design and to ensure that sample and effect sizes are sufficient to provide statistically significant evidence of change in the issue under investigation, and that the change is due to the intervention.

The major methods appropriate for injury prevention evaluation are summarized in Table 1. Each of these methods is outlined below and is illustrated by a relevant example from the international injury prevention literature.

Table 1. Evaluation methods for injury prevention interventions.

Randomized controlled trials
—individual randomization
—cluster randomization
Controlled trials (non-randomized)
Natural experiments
Case control studies
Time series modelling

What are randomized controlled trials (RCTs)?

Randomized controlled trials are experimental studies where participants or groups of participants are randomly assigned to an intervention group or to a control group. More than one intervention group can be used in such a study to determine the effectiveness of several counter-measures. This method is widely used in drug trials, where the control group may receive placebos.

An effective example using randomization of individuals was described by Miller et al (1982) where paediatrician counselling was provided and smoke detectors at cost price were available to the intervention group, in a RCT involving 120 well children in each of the intervention and control groups. A significant increase in detectors installed in the intervention households was observed compared with the control group where no change was observed.

Cluster randomization is a method of RCT where randomization occurs in clusters, such as local groups of intervention schools compared with control clusters. This method requires larger sample sizes and statistical correction for the effects of clustering. No effective examples using this methodology were identified in a comprehensive review of the child and adolescent literature on injury prevention by Towner et al (1996).

What are controlled trials?

These evaluations are usually conducted where RCTs are not possible and they are non-randomized. The method is said to be quasi-experimental. Here the control or comparison group is matched with the intervention group on a number of relevant variables to minimize differences in response to all other potentially confounding factors, and differences are observed over time.

The use of the term control or comparison group is dependent on the level of rigour that is achievable. Communities are generally more appropriately described as comparison groups since they are less homogenous and fewer factors can be matched than for individuals.

It is not possible to be certain that the comparison group's response to all other factors is the same as that of the target group. Multiple intervention and comparison groups enhance the evidence, but pose practical problems for the programme, particularly in terms of the resources required.

The Shire of Bulla Safe Living Programme (Hennessy et al, 1994) implemented 113 injury prevention strategies during a 3-year intervention period and the effects were compared with the Shire of Melton and the State of Victoria. Process, impact and injury outcome evaluation was conducted. The programme was shown to be partially effective. While no significant reduction in overall injury rates was shown, there was some evidence from pre- and post-intervention surveys of a reduction in minor injuries. Examples of hazard reductions were observed, such as greater than 50% implementation of more than 400 recommendations of a schools safety audit. Increased use of safety devices and safety equipment were also reported (Ozanne-Smith et al, 1994).

Multiple controls were used in a study of the effectiveness of a community-based injury prevention programme, undertaken by Guyer et al (1989), where five interventions (burns, poisoning, falls, suffocation and vehicle occupant) for children under 5 years were implemented in nine communities with five control communities, over a 2-year period. Effectiveness was demonstrated for vehicle occupant injuries in the intervention compared with control communities, but not for other elements of the programme.

How can meta analysis contribute?

Where sound research methods are used and results clearly reported in the published literature, the potential to obtain a meaningful overview of research findings and increased statistical power from a pool of controlled studies using comparable methods, is possible using meta-analysis. Here the evidence is reviewed by applying standard statistical analysis methods to all of the available studies that meet the selection criteria, with the potential to enhance the utility of the results. Few child injury prevention studies have yet been reported using this method.

Using the related method of a systematic review, Roberts et al (1996) reviewed randomized controlled trials of home visiting as an intervention for injury prevention in order to quantify their effectiveness. Here the method involved the systematic review of 11 RCTs of home visiting programmes, involving a total of 3433 participants. Pooled odds ratios were estimated as an inverse variance weighted average of the study-specific odds ratios. The results showed that, for the eight programmes that addressed the prevention of child injury, the pooled odds ratio was 0.74 (95% confidence interval 0.60–0.92). The authors concluded that home visiting programmes have the potential to reduce significantly the incidence of child injury.

What are natural experiments?

Opportunistic use can be made of natural experiments, where an intervention is implemented in one region but not in another, resulting in the availability of a control.

A number of road safety studies have been undertaken when state regulations have differed, particularly where changes have occurred in both directions over time.

One such example is the mandatory requirement for motorcycle helmets being differentially implemented and repealed between states in the USA. Legislation was introduced in 49 states between 1975 and 1979 and 27 of these states later repealed the legislation. As a result the helmet wearing rates decreased and head injuries increased in those states that repealed the legislation compared with those that retained the legislation (National Committee for Injury Prevention and Control, 1989).

What are case control studies?

Case control studies are an efficient method of undertaking a controlled evaluation study since the cases are selected as the result of an injury. Controls who do not have the injury but share some other characteristics with the case are selected. Cases and controls are compared by means of the probability of exposure to a particular protective or risk factor. It is fundamentally important that the controls are from the same population as the cases.

A recently published example of a case control study addresses height and surfacing as risk factors for injury in falls from playground equipment (Chalmers et al, 1996). This study evaluated the effectiveness of the height and surfacing requirements of the New Zealand standard for playgrounds and playground equipment. Of 300 children who had fallen from playground equipment, 110 (cases) had sustained an injury that required medical attention and 190 (controls) had not sustained injury requiring medical attention.

The risk of injury being sustained in a fall was increased if the equipment failed to comply with the maximum fall height, surfacing or safe fall height requirements. Falls from heights in excess of 1.5 m increased the risk 4.1 times that of falls from 1.5 m or less. It was estimated that a 45% reduction in children attending emergency departments due to playground falls could be achieved if the maximum fall height was lowered to 1.5 m (Chalmers et al, 1996).

It should be noted that difficulties may arise in the interpretation of such case control studies. This is because (a) the population exposed and unexposed to the potentially protective or risk factor are those people who segregate themselves to these categories (i.e. not matched or allocated) and (b) because there is rarely any analysis of change in risk with change in protective exposure, as required for all other evaluation designs.

What is time series modelling?

The effect of an injury prevention programme on a chosen criterion is measured by the difference between:

- the level of that criterion (e.g. injuries in the target group) that actually occurred, following the implementation of the programme, and
- the level that was expected to occur, if there had been no programme (Cameron, 1995).

Experimental or comparison groups may be used to determine this difference, as may time series modelling. In their simplest form, time series analyses model pre-implementation injury frequencies as a function of time and extrapolate these models to estimate expected post-implementation levels.

A combination of modelling and comparison uses the above technique, but adjusted for the change in level of the comparison group compared with an extrapolation of its past injury levels. Here, co-variate analysis is used to explain changes in the injury level occurring due to other than programme effects. This method relies on the definition, inclusion and measurement of all other factors, apart from the programme (Cameron, 1995).

Finally, in a more sophisticated combination of modelling and comparison, co-variate analysis is undertaken in separate time series models for the actual injury levels for the programme and comparison groups. The difference gives the best estimate of the programme effect. The change in comparison group injury levels (apparent programme effect) accounts for unknown factors in the simpler modelling method (Cameron, 1995).

Time series models incorporating co-variates may be interrupted or un-interrupted. The model may also be fitted using traditional multiple regression techniques as well as more recent time series methods. Interrupted time series models, as an alternative to incorporating trend, seasonality and other time dependencies, model pre- and post-implementation injury frequencies together and then test the significance of the intervention terms (discontinuities) (Cameron, 1995).

Evaluations of the effectiveness of bicycle helmet legislation demonstrate this methodology. In Victoria, Australia, cycle helmet wearing became compulsory in 1990. Subsequent changes in cycling head injury mortality, morbidity and insurance claims, in observed cycle helmet wearing, and in cycling exposure were entered into a time series model. The attributable effect of helmet use was separated out from those due to concurrent reductions in cycling exposure and secular traffic safety trends that had also led to a general reduction in cyclist injuries compared to the pre-law period (Cameron et al, 1994).

Conclusion

As professional and public awareness of the dimensions and nature of injury as a public health problem increases, it is essential to systematic further development that the question 'what works to prevent injury?' can be answered.

REFERENCES

American Association for Automotive Medicine (1985) The Abbreviated Injury Scale. IL: American Association for Automotive Medicine.

Avery JG, Harper P & Ackroyd S (1990) Do we pay too dearly for our sport and leisure activities? *Public Health* **104**: 171–182.

Baker S, O'Neill B & Haddow W (1976) The Injury Severity Score: a method for describing patients with multiple injuries and evaluating emergency care. *Journal of Trauma* **14**: 187–196.

Breeze E, Trevor G & Wilmot A (1991) *Accidents for Which Medical Advice was Sought.* Series GHS no.20. London: HMSO.

Cameron, M. (1995) Impact evaluation. In Ozanne-Smith J (ed.) *Injury Research and Prevention: A Text,* pp. 261–266. Melbourne, Australia: Monash University Accident Research Centre (MUARC).

*Cameron M, Vulcan A, Finch C et al (1994) Mandatory bicycle helmet use following a decade of helmet promotion in Victoria, Australia—an evaluation. *Accident Analysis and Prevention* **26**: 325–337.

Chalmers D, Marshall D, Langley J et al (1996) Height and surfacing as risk factors for injury in falls from playground equipment: a case control study. *Injury Prevention* **2**: 98–104.

DiGuiseppi C, Roberts I & Li L (1997) Influence of changing travel patterns on child death rates from injury: trend analysis. *British Medical Journal* **314**: 710–713.

DoH (Department of Health) (1996a) *Hospital Episode Statistics. Volume 1—Finished Consultant Episodes by Diagnosis, Operation and Specialty. England: Financial year 1993–94.* London: HMSO.

DoH (Department of Health) (1996b) *Hospital Episode Statistics. Volume 2—Finished Consultant Episodes: injury/poisoning by external causes.* England: financial year 1993–94.

*DoT (Department of Transport) (1994) *Road Accidents Great Britain 1993. The Casualty Report.* London: HMSO.

Dowswell T, Jarvis S & Towner E (1994) Reducing childhood Accidents. The Effectiveness of Health Promotion Interventions: An Annotated Bibliography. Newcastle upon Tyne: Northern and Yorkshire Regional Health Authority.

*Drummond A & Ozanne-Smith J (1991) *The Behaviour and Crash Involvement Risk of Child Pedestrians and Bicyclists: A Traffic Exposure Study* (Report No. 17). Melbourne, Australia: Monash University Accident Research Centre (MUARC).

*DTI (Department of Trade and Industry) (1994) *Home and Leisure Accident Research. 1992 Data.* 16th Annual Report. London: DTI Consumer Safety Unit.

Guyer B, Gallagher S, Chang B et al (1989) Prevention of childhood injuries: evaluation of the Statewide Childhood Injury Prevention Program (SCIPP). *American Journal of Public Health* **79**: 1521–1527.

*Haddon W (1973) Energy damage and the ten countermeasure strategies. *Journal of Trauma* **13**: 321–331.

Hennessy M, Arnold R & Harvey P (1994) *The First Three Years: Final Report of the First Three Years of the Shire of Bulla's Safe Living Program (1991–1993).* Victoria: Monash University Accident Research Centre (MUARC).

Home Office (1992) *Summary Fire Statistics: United Kingdom 1991.* Home Office Statistical Bulletin Issue 27/92. London: Home Office.

HSE (Health and Safety Executive) (1995) *Health and Safety Statistics.* London: HMSO.

Jarvis S, Towner E & Walsh S (1996) Unintentional injury. In Botting B (ed.) *The Health of our Children: A Review in the Mid-1990's,* pp 95–112. London: Office of Population Censuses and Surveys.

Jones-Lee MW (1993) Personal willingness to pay for prevention: evaluating the consequences of accidents as a basis for preventive measures. *Addiction* **88**: 913–921.

Kraus J (1985) Effectiveness of measures to prevent unintentional deaths of infants and children from suffocation and strangulation. *Public Health Reports* **100**: 231–240.

Kujala U, Taimela S, Antti-Poika I et al (1995) Acute injuries in soccer, ice hockey, volleyball, basketball, judo and karate: analysis of national registry data. *British Medical Journal* **311:** 1465–1468.

Langley J (1982) The international classification of diseases codes for describing injuries and the circumstances surrounding injuries: a critical comment and suggestions for improvement. *Accident Analysis and Prevention* **14:** 195–197.

Levene S (1991) Coroners' records of accidental deaths. *Archives of Disease in Childhood* **66:** 1239–1241.

MacKenzie E (1984) Injury severity scales. *American Journal of Emergency Medicine* **2:** 537–549.

MacKenzie E (1996) Possibilities and problems with severity scaling for evaluation and research in the process of measuring the severity and costs of accidental injury. European Consumer Safety Association.

MacKenzie E, Steinwachs D, Shankar B et al (1986) An ICD-9CM to AIS Conversion Table: Development and Application. Paper presented at the 30th Annual Meeting of the American Association for Automotive Medicine, Montreal, Quebec.

Mackenzie J (1996) The Work of the Victoria State Traffic Accident Commission. Plenary Presentation. Paper presented at the 3rd International Conference on Injury Prevention and Control, Melbourne, Australia, February 1996.

Miller R, Reisinger K, Blatter M et al (1982) Pediatric counseling and subsequent use of smoke detectors. *American Journal of Public Health* **72:** 392–393.

Morgenstern H (1982) Uses of ecological analysis in epidemiological research. *American Journal of Public Health* **72:** 1136–1144.

*MUARC (Monash University Accident Research Centre, University of Melbourne) (1993–1997) VISS data collection system. *Hazard* **1** (all copies relevant).

Mynors P & Savell A (1992) *Cycling on the Continent.* London: Local Authority Cycle Planning Group.

National Committee for Injury Prevention and Control (1989) *Injury Prevention: meeting the Challenge.* New York: Oxford University Press.

*ONS (Office for National Statistics) (1997a) *1995 Mortality Statistics: Childhood, Infant and Perinatal England and Wales.* Series DH3 No. 28. London: HMSO.

ONS (Office for National Statistics (1997b) *1995 Mortality Statistics by cause England and Wales.* Series DH 2. London: HMSO.

OPCS (Office of Population Censuses and Surveys) (1988) *Occupational Mortality: Childhood Supplement. Registrar General's Decennial Supplement for England and Wales, 1979–80, 1982–83.* Vol. 8. London: HMSO.

OPCS (Office of Population Censuses and Surveys) (1991) *Small Area Statistics—1991 Census of the Population of England and Wales.* London: HMSO.

OPCS (Office of Population Censuses and Surveys) (1993) *Mortality Statistics: Fatal Accidents Occuring during sports and Leisure Activities.* London: HMSO.

Ozanne-Smith J, Sherrard J, Brumen I et al (1994) *Community Based Injury Prevention Evaluation Report: Shire of Bulla Safe Living Program* Report No. 66. Melbourne, Australia: Monash University Accident Research Centre (MUARC).

Peterson L, Harbeck C & Moreno A (1993) Measures of children's injuries: self-reported versus maternal-reported events with temporally proximal versus delayed reporting. *Journal of Pediatric Psychology* **18:** 133–147.

Reading R & Openshaw S (1993) Do inaccuracies in small deprivation analyses matter? *Journal of Epidemiology and Community Health* **14:** 195–197.

Roberts I, Kramer M & Suissa S (1996) Does home visiting prevent childhood injury? A systematic review of randomised controlled trials. *British Medical Journal* **312:** 29–33.

Robertson L (1980) Crash involvement of teenaged drivers when driver education is eliminated from high school. *American Journal of Public Health* **70:** 599–605.

Royal College of General Practitioners & OPCS (1995) *Morbidity Statistics from General Practice: Fourth National Study 1991–1992.* London: HMSO.

Schelp L (1988) The role of organizations in community participation—prevention of accidental injuries in a rural Swedish municipality. *Social Science and Medicine* **26:** 1087–1093.

*Sharples P, Storey A, Aynsley-Green A et al (1990a) Avoidable factors contributing to death of children with head injury. *British Medical Journal* **300:** 87–91.

Sharples P, Storey A, Aynsley-Green A et al (1990b) Causes of fatal childhood accidents involving head injury in Northern region, 1979–86. *British Medical Journal* **301:** 1193–1197.

*Sherrard J (1995) Issues in program evaluation. In Ozanne-Smith J (ed.) *Injury Research and Prevention: A Text*, pp. 2581–2611. Melbourne, Australia: Monash University Accident Research Centre (MUARC).

Towner E, Jarvis S, Walsh S et al (1994) Measuring exposure to injury risk in schoolchildren aged 11–14. *British Medical Journal* **308:** 449–452.

*Towner E, Dowswell T, Simpson G et al (1996) *Health Promotion in Childhood and Young Adolescence for the Prevention of Unintentional Injuries*, Vol. 1. London: Health Education Authority.

Vulcan A, Cameron M & Watson W (1992) Mandatory bicycle helmet use: experience in Victoria, Australia. *World Journal of Surgery* **16:** 389–397.

Walsh S, Jarvis S, Towner E et al (1996) Annual incidence of unintentional injury among 54 000 children. *Injury Prevention* **2:** 16–20.

Walton W (1982) An evaluation of the Poison Prevention Packaging Act. *Pediatrics* **69:** 363–370.

Yates D & Woodford M (1992) First report of the UK Major Trauma Outcome Study. *British Medical Journal* **305:** 737–740.

2

Causes and prevention of home injuries

MICHAEL HAYES BSc, PhD

Projects Director

SARA LEVENE MA, MB BChir, MRCP, MRCPCH

Medical Consultant

Child Accident Prevention Trust, Clerk's Court, 18–20 Farringdon Lane, London EC1R 3AU, UK

Accidents and unintentional injuries in the home are closely related to the normal behaviour of children, their exposure to hazards and deprivation. The classic approaches to prevention are education, engineering and legislation. In addition, families can, to a greater or lesser extent, use supervision of the child to minimize risk of injury. Priorities for prevention can be defined in several ways but for the family it is likely that preventing serious and fatal injuries will be the main concern. The most important home accidents in terms of death and injury are house fires and other thermal injuries, falls, drownings, poisoning, choking, suffocation and entrapment and glass lacerations. This chapter reviews preventive approaches for these types of accidents, highlighting those that are known to be effective.

Key words: accident; injury; home; baby; child; prevention.

Accidental injury in the home is preventable. Understanding the underlying causes leads to understanding what prevention measures to try and at whom they should be directed. Some preventative measures have been evaluated and some have been demonstrated to be effective (Towner et al, 1996).

The use in the text of the word 'accident' does not imply the consequence of an unpredictable irremediable situation.

CAUSES OF HOME INJURIES

Primary factors

A number of factors underlie the large number of home accidents. Some are primary and others are secondary exacerbating factors. The most basic factor is the normal behaviour of children. Children are less experienced than adults and more likely to be impulsive and experimental (Berfenstam, 1977). With time children mature in their intellectual and social skills. As children develop increased physical skills and as they grow in size, the physical expression of their behaviour also changes.

An understanding of normal child development is therefore fundamental to understanding how accidents happen to children of different ages (Jackson, 1977). A simple example is that of falls. The newborn infant is only able to fall if dropped by a carer or a sibling. As the child develops more vigorous movements, they may fall if placed high up. They can make a bouncing cradle fall from a work surface or table, they can roll over and fall from a changing table or bed. Once the child can crawl, they can crawl onto furniture or up stairs and then fall down. A babywalker provided at this age will give much increased mobility with the potential for falls over thresholds or down steps (Kavanagh and Banco, 1982). The walking child will fall on the level and may injure themselves on low furniture or low lying glass. The more skilled climber who has the manual dexterity to open a window may fall out from a height. The older child who is allowed to explore the yard or garden may climb and fall from a high wall or a tree. Different preventative measures are relevant for all these circumstances (see Table 1).

Another simple primary factor is exposure. Younger children spend time at home rather than in school, in the leisure environment or on the roads. Younger children are therefore over-represented in home accident statistics. Exposure also predicts other features, for example the rooms in which more injuries take place (DTI, 1997).

Boys are more at risk of injury and death in the home than girls (Woodruffe et al, 1993; DTI, 1997).

Secondary factors

The home should provide a safe setting for the children. Their homes should be designed to enhance their safety and reduce the number of hazards to which they are exposed (Sinnott, 1985).

However, children are placed at risk because the environment of the home is designed with the needs of the adult and not those of the child in mind. More often, these are the aesthetic needs of the adult. This leads to the presence of features such as horizontal banisters, which a child may climb over; a wood burning stove in the centre of a room in a prize winning house design (Rowland, 1996); low level glass in doors to patios or within the house. There may also be conflicts between features intended to increase safety for older people and the safety of young children, for example waist level sockets are readily accessible to children as well as to the elderly.

Another very important factor is deprivation. There is a very clear relationship between the incidence of accidental childhood injury and indicators of deprivation such as socio-economic class. In childhood, the gradient for accidental death with respect to social class is more marked that for any other cause (Woodruffe et al, 1993). It is becoming more steep,

Table 1. Safety and child development.

Accident	Age and stage						
	Newborn wriggling, rolling	Sitting and reaching	Crawling and walking	2 years	3 years	5 years	8 years
Falls	Dropping baby Falling with baby	Dropping off changing table Babywalker—may lead to falls and bumps	Crawls and falls on stairs **Stairgate** Falls out—buggy, high-chair **Harnesses**	Windows Window catches	Climbing and playing Climbs out of cot	Garden toys	Playground
Cuts and bruises		Sharp objects on ground	Glass doors and windows **Safety film on glass**		Sharp objects in house **Catches on drawers**	Sharp objects in garage	Hobbies, cooking
Burns and scalds	**Smoke detector** Bathwater too hot Feeds too hot	Reaches for hot cups and food	Crawls into fires, radiators **Fireguards** Pulls kettle flex **Coiled flex**	Uses matches, lighters **Cupboard catches**			Hobbies, cooking
Swallowing and choking	Unsupervised feeding Cords around neck—never tie on dummy	Cleaners and medicines left out Clutter on floor like buttons or screws	Open cupboard doors **Cupboard catches** Older children's toys	Pots and packets without child resistant caps; plastic bags **Catches on drawers**		Probably manages peanuts	
Road and car	**Rear facing baby carrier**		**Reins in the street Second stage car seat**		Learn pavement is for people, road is for cars	**Booster cushion** Learn to stop and wait for adult at kerb	Cycle helmet Cycle training Green Cross Code **Adult lap and shoulder belt**
Drowning	Drowning in bath			Drowning in ponds		Swimming lessons	May swim with friends at pool but beware open water

Source: Child Accident Prevention Trust, 1992.

as falls in mortality are larger in upper social classes (Roberts and Power, 1996)

The explanation is not so clear cut. It is not that people living in poverty do not care for their children and wish them to be safe. Rather, the circumstances in which they live present the children with far more physical hazards. Money is not available to make essential repairs or to buy safety equipment. Landlords may obstruct alterations essential for child safety. Reactive depression is almost a natural consequence of the environment, and the depressed parent may be simply unable to provide their child with the supervision and support that the environment demands. In these circumstances, it is perhaps more useful to ask why accident numbers are not even higher, and to commend parents for keeping their children safe (Roberts et al, 1995).

PREVENTATIVE APPROACHES

Much injury prevention literature uses technical headings for approaches to child injury prevention. These are education, engineering and enforcement (Child Accident Prevention Trust, 1989).

Education is the giving of injury prevention training or advice. This may be directed at the general public, through individual or small group approaches, or through wider publicity campaigns. It may be directed at professionals in their training or their continued professional development, be it health workers or others who may affect child safety directly such as architects or planners.

Mass media campaigns and interventions aimed at the general population are at best partially effective. Community wide prevention programmes as pioneered in Scandinavia and America have now been documented in many settings. These programmes attempt to change community attitudes to accidents and increase resources that facilitate prevention. Evaluations are rarely randomized controlled trials, but the cumulative effects of a number of evaluations suggest that this approach is of value (Schelp, 1987; Guyer et al, 1989; Banbury, 1992; Davidson et al, 1994). The key to this approach is the formation of healthy alliances, where health professionals combine with those from other fields to improve child safety (Towner et al, 1996)

Engineering is the design of products or the built environment to minimize the potential for accidental injury. This may mean the provision of special safety features (impact absorbent surfaces, safety products). However, it is more important to undertake risk assessment as part of the development of any product line and so eliminate potentially hazardous features. The removal of hazardous features has been demonstrated to reduce the incidence of injuries related to consumer products (Sorensen, 1976).

Enforcement is the use of regulation or legislation to reinforce safety practices. Examples in domestic safety in the UK are control of nightwear flammability and the mandatory use of child resistant closures on certain products. The latter has been shown to lead to a reduction in admissions for accidental poisoning (DoH, 1975; Jackson, 1983).

Home safety is actually achieved by the domestic strategies of families. These may include education, explaining things to children and training them. This may fail because children do not understand the message or choose to ignore it. Engineering is also a possibility, with the separation of the child from hazards by improvements in the environment or the fitting and use of safety equipment. This strategy depends on parental knowledge, practical skill and finances.

Families may also employ supervision as a strategy. This may be the only possibility in some circumstances such as preventing infants from drowning in the bath. It may break down because it is too demanding and the circumstances in which close supervision is needed are not fully appreciated (Levene, 1996; Roberts, 1996)

Interventions within the family must be sensitive to the needs of the family and their current knowledge and success with respect to safety. Strategies must be sensitive to the needs of the families rather than based on what the professionals think is best (Roberts, 1996). Carefully planned education can be effective (Colver et al, 1982). Social support to counteract isolation and depression as well as to provide advice on parenting may be of value. Roberts and Pless (1995) highlight the particular needs of single mothers.

PRIORITIES FOR PREVENTION

Priorities are likely to be based on the combination of a number of factors including, for example:

- Types of injuries—those that are most likely to cause death or disability, the most frequent, the most expensive in terms of treatment, those for which effective prevention strategies exist.
- Types of accidents—those for which effective prevention strategies exist, those that can be addressed by the individual rather than the authorities, the most frequent, etc.
- Skills, knowledge and attitudes of those responsible for implementing the intervention, whether the person be a practitioner or a parent.
- Availability of resources for prevention—including financial and staffing.
- Political climate—for example, different priorities may exist depending on whether the government supports a deregulatory approach or not.
- Timescale for implementation of the intervention.
- Presence or absence of a strategic framework or policy.

In the context of accidents in the home, the preventive measures are highly likely to be within the control of the parent so a number of the considerations outlined above become less important. The key points for a parent will probably be to prevent accidents that are likely to cause serious injury and death, albeit with cost considerations being relevant. Analysis of statistical information on accidents and injuries points towards the following topics as being most important:

- House fires and other thermal injuries.
- Falls.
- Drownings.
- Poisoning.
- Choking, suffocation and entrapments.
- Glass injuries.

These are dealt with in detail below.

Electrocution and injuries from toys are often perceived by the public as presenting particular hazards to children but both are already well controlled or do not, in reality, result in significant numbers or severity of injury.

Electricity can clearly present hazards but within the home environment it is fire from electrical appliances or poor wiring that is the cause of death and injury, rather than electrocution. The design of electrical sockets in the UK makes it very difficult for children to gain access to live contacts as a probe has to be inserted into the earth hole in order to open the others. The other danger that can arise is due to children plugging in electrical appliances, especially irons and heaters, which can either lead to contact burns or house fires. There is no evidence that plug-in socket covers, which are readily available and widely used, are effective.

Many aspects of toy design, including mechanical properties, accessibility of small parts and sharp points and edges, flammability, toxicity, stability and entrapment hazards are tightly controlled by a mandatory European standard, BS EN 71 (British Standards Institution, 1988). In addition, toys are required to carry warnings about their suitability or otherwise for certain age groups, especially when they may present a hazard to children under 36 months. Even well designed and constructed toys can present two specific risks: use by children for which they were not intended resulting particularly in choking hazards, and as precipitators of falls when left lying around the house, most seriously on staircases. The former problem can be addressed through public education linked with clearly understood labelling but cannot be eliminated in households containing children of a wide age range. The latter problem is more difficult to address as its remedy requires a change of behaviour of children and their parents.

House fires and other thermal injuries

House fires are the leading cause of death among children in the home. The contribution that they make to the total varies according to the age of the children. Overall, for children under 15 years, house fires ranked second to road accidents as a cause of accidental death, constituting 12% of accidental deaths. The age dependency reflects the fact that babies are completely dependent on adults for assistance in a house fire, being incapable of helping themselves, and that young children, who may be able to escape, tend to seek safety within the home and hence suffer the adverse consequences. For older children they rank first or second depending on the year reviewed. There have been downward trends in the numbers of fire deaths for each of the age groups with the decline being most marked among children aged under 5 years. For babies under 1 year, the 1994 total was less than 30% of the 1986 peak and for children aged 1–4 years the 34 deaths in 1994 under half of the worst year (1987). However, trends in deaths per million population among the under ones and 1–4 year olds show significant declines but less than for the raw numbers.

Data from the British Crime Survey (Home Office, 1995) showed that single parent families had the highest risk of having a fire in their homes, while risks for households with children were greater than for those without. Poor condition of the housing was also identified as presenting a high risk of fire.

Three topics are of particular note in the context of preventing death and injury in house fires. There have been a number of studies of interventions aimed at increasing smoke alarm use as a means of reducing casualties but most have been methodologically flawed or have produced inconclusive results (see Towner et al, 1996 for a full discussion). A study in Oklahoma City (Mallonee et al 1996), however, does indicate that a targeted intervention involving a smoke alarm give-away programme can reduce the incidence of injuries from residential fires.

Smokers' materials (tobacco products, matches and lighters) are cited as a frequent cause of fires in the home. Within this group of materials, cigarette lighters pose a special risk as they are often capable of being operated by children. There are now requirements in some countries, notably the USA, Canada and Australia, for lighters to be child resistant. However, the adequacy of the requirements and their enforcement is open to question. No similar requirements currently exist in the European Union (Jenkins, 1996; Lant, 1996).

One of the main causes of death in house fires is the toxic smoke that is given off by burning upholstered furniture. Regulations exist in the UK (DTI, 1988) that ban the most hazardous grades of foam in furniture. In 1992, the regulations were extended to cover second-hand furniture and furniture in holiday homes. Home Office data reveal that the number of deaths per 1000 fires where the item mainly responsible for the fire was upholstered furniture fell from 51 in 1988 to 34 in 1991, although it has stabilized at about 40 subsequently (Home Office, 1995).

Scalds are also a frequent cause of thermal injury to children. Two causes that have been the focus of particular preventive action are the lowering of the temperature of tap water and the use of coiled flexes for electric kettles. There is evidence that the legislative approach and a broadly based campaign to reduce tap water temperature can reduce both the number of child scald casualties and the water temperature (Erdmann et al, 1991; Waller et al, 1993). A frequent cause of accidents involving kettles has been children reaching up and pulling kettle flexes that overhang the edge of work surfaces but no evaluation has been reported on the use of coiled or short kettle flexes as a means of reducing associated injuries.

Falls

A large proportion of the injuries that children suffer in the home are falls. The Department of Trade and Industry report that in 1995, 42% of the under fives who attended hospital following unintentional injuries had suffered falls, while for 5–14 year olds the figure was 35% (DTI, 1997). Many of the falls are simply trips and stumbles (termed 'falls on the same level') or occur on stairs with very few being fatal.

Safety gates, for which there is a British Standard, BS 4125: 1991 (British Standards Institution, 1991), are frequently used to prevent falls on stairs but their effectiveness has not been evaluated in the home. The standard requires them to withstand impacts by a 2 year old child running into them and outlaws designs that could be easily climbed over by young children. The appropriateness of using the equivalent of a 2 year old to test safety gates is open to question as research in the UK has shown that children up to 4 years cannot negotiate stairs reliably (Nixon et al, 1987).

Falls from windows and balconies are more serious in their consequences. A community wide campaign in New York (Speigel and Lindaman, 1977) provided window guards to 4200 families in order to prevent falls. The intervention reduced window falls by over 30% and associated mortality by 35%. Devices are available to restrict the opening of windows without adult supervision to 100 mm but these are not required under UK Building Regulations. Small children can squeeze through larger gaps. There is a need to balance two safety issues—the need to prevent falls and allow escape in a fire.

The prevention of falls from balconies is addressed within the Building Regulations (Department of the Environment and the Welsh Office, 1991), which include requirements that balconies should not be climbable and the guarding should prevent children passing through. The regulations recommend that the guarding height should be at least 1100 mm. Falls from domestic balconies have been analysed in a pamphlet from the Building Research Establishment (Webber and Aizlewood, 1993).

Drowning

For young children, drownings occur in the domestic environment (Kemp and Sibert, 1992). The location of the event reflects strongly the range of mobility of the child, with those involving babies tending to occur in the bath, and toddlers being drowned in garden ponds or domestic swimming pools, especially those of neighbours. A problem reported frequently in the USA is drowning in large buckets (Mann et al, 1992).

The prevention of drownings to babies relies heavily on parent education (Colver and Pearson, 1985), emphasizing the need for constant supervision when the baby is in water. Fences with self-locking gates can reduce the risk of drownings for toddlers in domestic swimming pools. Above-ground, rather than in-ground pools, can also affect the numbers of drownings (see Towner et al, 1996, pp. 46–47, for a full discussion of this topic).

Poisoning

Poisoning, or more correctly, suspected poisoning is the cause of large numbers of visits for young children to accident and emergency departments. The Department of Trade and Industry Home Accident Surveillance System reveals that over 36 000 children made such visits in 1995 (DTI 1997).

The use of child-resistant packaging for drugs has been shown to be beneficial (Sibert et al, 1977, Palmisano, 1981, Walton, 1982) although not perfect by any means (Sibert et al, 1985). The use of poison labels, such as Mr Yuk stickers, as a means of preventing poisoning has been shown to be ineffective (Fergusson et al, 1982).

Many poisoning incidents are caused by products other than drugs. In the UK, a specified list of common, hazardous household chemicals are required to be sold in child-resistant containers although the effectiveness of the regulations has not been evaluated. However, the use of child-resistant containers for the storage of paraffin in South Africa has been shown to be effective (Krug et al, 1994).

Choking, suffocation and entrapment

For children under 5 years, choking, suffocation and entrapment pose major hazards. Food, small objects, including toys or parts of toys, nursery furniture, especially bunk beds, cots and mattresses, and anything with cords attached can injure or kill babies and toddlers. It is normal behaviour for children under 3 years to put things in their mouths. For babies, entrapment between the mattress and the side of the cot can be highly dangerous.

Bunk beds that contain gaps in their framework that allow a child's body to pass through but not their head are also exceptionally dangerous and are covered by regulation in the UK. Toys that are small or include small parts are regarded as unsuitable for children under 3 years and have to be labelled as such. The test for size is whether or not the toy will fit into a so-called truncated cylinder but this test is the subject of some criticism. British and international standards exist for the ventilation of pen caps developed following the deaths of a number of children in the 4–15 year age range, not the ages normally associated with inhalation deaths.

Curtain and blind cords, dangling electric flexes, cords in clothing and attached to toys, especially cot toys, can and have all led to strangulation.

Glass injuries

Glass is widely used architecturally and in furniture as well as in containers. Its danger is well recognized when used as a container, especially when already broken, but its threat of severe and fatal injury in its other guises is less obvious, not only for children.

Safety glass—glass that either does not break readily or may break but into less injurious fragments—is now required under Building Regulations in new housing in the UK for low level glazing and in other potentially hazardous locations. Common prevention strategies include replacing dangerous glass either with unglazed panels or safety glass, or covering the glass with a clear plastic film.

In furniture, there are deaths on record from children falling through glass tables, resulting in lacerations and death due to loss of blood. To address potentially dangerous tables, a British Standard, BS 7376, has been published (British Standards Institution, 1990).

CONCLUSIONS

It is impossible to prevent all unintentional injuries, whether in the home or elsewhere, without the expenditure of greater resources than are available or through restrictions on childrens' and adults' lives that would be socially unacceptable. Allowing children to suffer injuries as part of 'growing up' or a learning process cannot be condoned. However, taking risks in controlled situations is beneficial to children's development. The home should be a place of comfort and safety for children where they are able to develop to their full potential without the risk of severe injury.

REFERENCES

Banbury J (1992) *Play it Safe. Evaluation of Broadcasts and Back up Material*. London: BBC.

Berfenstam R (1977) The work of the Swedish joint committee for accident prevention. In Jackson RH (ed.) *Children, The Environment and Accidents*, pp. 141–153. Tunbridge: Pitman Medical

British Standards Institution (1988) *BS EN 71 Safety of Toys*. London: BSI.

British Standards Institution (1990) *BS 7376 Specification for the Inclusion of Glass in the Construction of Tables or Trolleys*. London: BSI.

British Standards Institution (1991) *BS 4125 Specification for Safety Requirements for Child Safety Barriers for Domestic Use*. London: BSI.

*Child Accident Prevention Trust (1989) *Basic Principles of Child Accident Prevention*. London: Child Accident Prevention Trust.

Child Accident Prevention Trust (1992) *Accident Prevention in Day Care and Play Settings: A Practical Guide*. London: Child Accident Prevention Trust.

Colver A & Pearson P (1985) Safety in the home. How well are we doing? *Health Visitor* 58: 41–42.

Colver A, Hutchinson P & Judson E (1982) Promoting children's home safety. *British Medical Journal* 285: 1177–1180.

Davidson LL, Durkin MS, Kuhn L et al (1994) The impact of safe kids/healthy neighbourhoods injury prevention program in Harlem, 1988 through 1991. *American Journal of Public Health* 84: 580–586.

Department of the Environment and the Welsh Office (1991) *The Building Regulations Approved Document K Stairs, Ramps and Guards* 1992 (edn). London: HMSO.

DoH (Department of Health) (1975) *Medicines (Child Safety) Regulations 1975*. London: HMSO.

DTI (Department of Trade and Industry) (1988) *Furniture and Furnishings (Fire Safety) Regulations 1988*. London: HMSO.

*DTI (Department of Trade and Industry) (1997) *Home Accident Surveillance System Annual Report 1995*. London: Department of Trade and Industry.

Erdmann T, Feldman K, Rivara F et al (1991) Tap water burn prevention: the effect of legislation. *Pediatrics* 88: 572–577.

Fergusson DM, Horwood LJ, Beautrais AL et al (1982) A controlled field trial of poisoning prevention methods. *Pediatrics* 69: 515–520.

*Guyer B, Gallagher S, Chang B et al (1989) Prevention of childhood injuries: evaluation of the Statewide Childhood Injury Prevention Program (SCIPP). *American Journal of Public Health* **79:** 1521–1527.

Home Office (1995) *Fire Statistics United Kingdom 1993*. London: Home Office.

Jackson RH (1977) Setting the scene. In Jackson RH (ed.) *Children, The Environment and Accidents*, pp 1–4. Tunbridge: Pitman Medical.

Jackson RH (1983) Childhood poisoning: perspectives and problems. *Human Toxicology* **2:** 285–293.

Jenkins D (1996) Bargain lighters can kill. *Trading Standards Review* **104:** 14–15.

Kavanagh CA & Banco L (1982) The infant walker: a previously unrecognized health hazard. *American Journal of Disease in Childhood* **136:** 205–206.

Kemp A & Sibert J (1992) Drowning and near-drowning in the United Kingdom: lessons for prevention. *British Medical Journal* **304:** 1143–1146.

Krug A, Ellis JB, Hay IT et al (1994) The impact of child resistant containers in the incidence of paraffin (kerosene) ingestion in children. *South African Medical Journal* **84:** 730–734.

Lant DP (1996) Bargain lighters can kill. *Trading Standards Review* **104:** 26–27.

*Levene S (1996) Is there more to parental supervision than political incorrectness? *Injury Prevention* **2:** 10–11.

Mallonee S, Istre GR, Rosenberg M et al (1996) Surveillance and prevention of residential-fire injuries. *New England Journal of Medicine* **335:** 27–31.

Mann CN, Weller S & Rauchschwalbe R (1992) Bucket-related drownings in the United States, 1984 through 1990. *Pediatrics* **89:** 1068–1071.

Nixon J, Jackson RH & Hayes HRM (1987) *An Analysis of Childhood Falls Involving Stairs and Bannisters*. London: Department of Trade and Industry.

Palmisano PA (1981). Targeted intervention in the control of drug overdoses by children. *Public Health Reports* **96:** 151–156.

*Roberts H, Smith SJ & Bryce C (1995) *Children at Risk? Safety As a Social Value*. Buckingham: Open University Press.

*Roberts I (1996) Parental supervision: a popular myth. *Injury Prevention* **2:** 9–10.

Roberts I & Pless B (1995) Social policy as a cause of childhood accidents: the children of lone mothers. *British Medical Journal* **311:** 925–928.

Roberts I & Power C (1996) Does the decline in child injury mortality vary by social class? A comparison of class specific mortality in 1981 and 1991. *British Medical Journal* **313:** 784–786.

Rowland T (1996) *Daily Telegraph* (London) August 17.

*Schelp L (1987) Community intervention and changes in accident pattern in a rural Swedish municipality. *Health Promotion* **2:** 109–125.

Sibert JR, Craft AW & Jackson RH (1977) Child resistant packaging and accidental child poisoning. *Lancet* **ii:** 289–290.

Sibert JR, Clarke AJ & Mitchell MP (1985) Improvements in child resistant containers. *Archives of Disease in Childhood* **60:** 1155–1157.

Sinnott R (1985) *Safety and Security in Building Design*. London: Collins.

Sorensen B (1976) The prevention of burns and scalds in a developed country. *Journal of Trauma* **16:** 249–258.

Speigel C & Lindaman F (1977) Children can't fly: a program to prevent childhood morbidity and mortality from window falls. *American Journal of Public Health* **67:** 1143–1147.

*Towner E, Dowsell T, Simpson G & Jarvis S (1996) *Health Promotion in Childhood and Adolescence for the Prevention of Unintentional Injuries*. London: Health Education Authority.

Waller AE, Clark J & Langley JD (1993) An evaluation of a program to reduce home tap water temperatures. *American Journal of Public Health* **17:** 116–123.

Walton W (1982) An evaluation of the Poison Prevention Packaging Act. *Pediatrics* **69:** 363–370.

Webber GMB & Aizlewood CE (1993) *Falls from Domestic Balconies. BRE Information Paper IP18/93*. Watford: Building Research Establishment.

*Woodruffe C, Glickman M, Barker M & Power C (1993) *Children, Teenagers and Health: The Key Data*. Buckingham: Open University Press.

3

Causes and prevention of leisure, school and work injuries

JO R. SIBERT MA, MB BChir, DCH, DObst, RCOG, MD, FRCP, FRCPCH
Professor of Community Child Health
Department of Child Health, University of Wales College of Medicine, 1st Floor, Academic Centre, Llandough Hospital, Cardiff, South Glamorgan CF64 2XX, UK

JIM NIXON BSocWk, MSocWk, BA, PhD
Senior Lecturer in Medical Social Work
Department of Child Health, University of Queensland, Royal Children's Hospital, Herston, Queensland 4029, Australia

Injuries to children provide a major challenge for analysis and prevention. Play is vital for the children in their physical development and their ability to make social relationships. Recent research suggests that attention to the surface and height of play equipment should reduce injuries in public playgrounds. All forms of sport and recreation have some risk but with attention, injuries can be prevented.

Drowning continues to be a major cause of death among children throughout the world. Injury rates in municipal swimming pools are low, but rates in domestic pools appear to be high. Drowning in rivers, canals and lakes is predominantly a problem of older boys playing unsupervised.

The UN Convention on the Rights of the Child stresses the right for protection from work which is harmful to the child's health. There is clear evidence that some children are at particular risk of injuries, including on farms.

INJURIES AT PLAY

Play is vital for children in their physical development and their ability to develop social relationships. Clearly there is always the potential for injury to the child in play. Toys are an important component of many aspects of play. However despite much concern there is little evidence that they seriously harm children. Only one child died in England and Wales in a 2 year period by inhaling a toy (Nixon et al, 1995). This is probably because of the firm toy safety regulations in Europe and other parts of the developed world. Although children do play at home and in organized groups (Sacks et al, 1990), many play in playgrounds provided by local authorities and private organizations. Much of the concern regarding injuries to children has been focused on potential problems in playgrounds. They provide an alternative to playing in dangerous places such as the road and need to be as safe as possible. Playgrounds were originally developed to offer play opportunities in an increasingly industrialized society during the nineteenth century (Heseltine and Holborn, 1987). Their safety is important not only in prevention of injuries but also because families need the assurance that it is safe for their children to play.

Playground Injuries

Public playground provision, safety and maintenance in Britain and in many other parts of the developed world are largely the responsibility of the local Councils. In Britain there has been much work in developing safer equipment and surfaces and in producing acceptable safety standards (BS 5696 and BS 7188: Heseltine et al, 1989). However these standards have largely been developed in the laboratory (Lewis et al, 1993) and there has been little analysis of real children having real injuries on real playgrounds (Sacks et al, 1990). Impact absorbing surfaces have been introduced to lessen the severity of a head injury from falling from equipment onto a hard surface. These may be either bark, sand or special impact absorbing rubberized tiles. However recent criticisms of these surfaces include a lack of proven studies of their effectiveness and their high cost (Ball and King, 1991).

Injuries to children in playgrounds

Illingworth et al (1975) studied children with a variety of playground injuries, and found that fractures were three times more common in this group than attendances in accident and emergency departments as a whole. The Leisure Accident Surveillance System (LASS) estimates that there are 24 000 playground injuries each half year in England and Wales (MacCleary, 1989). Mott et al (1994) reviewed playground injuries in a single city: they found 1.5% of hospital attendances were due to injuries sustained in a playground. They also found children injured on public playgrounds have a higher hospital admission rate and fracture rate compared to other types of injury. A few children die each year in playground accidents. Fourteen deaths occurred in Brisbane during play and recreation over a 5 year period (Nixon et al, 1981). None of these studies related injuries to the numbers of children playing.

Factors in Playground Design and Injuries

Information on playground injuries to children is clearly vital for those who produce safety standards and equipment and those who plan playgrounds for children. The safety of children on public playgrounds is a complex interaction between a number of factors (Mott et al, 1994):

- Type of equipment.
- Type of surface.
- Height of equipment.
- Numbers children playing.
- Type of play.
- Maintenance of the surface.
- Maintenance of the equipment.
- Weather.
- Supervision.

These factors are interlinked and the playground should be considered as a whole when preventive strategies are attempted. Reliable exposure data in the analysis of playground accident data is clearly important. Mott et al (1996, 1997) have developed a method of measuring exposure of children to play injuries relying on the observations of the people who work on the playgrounds.

Safety surfacing

Safety surfacing is protective against injuries to children on playgrounds (Mott et al, 1996). Its installation alone is insufficient however to prevent all injuries to children and children were not protected by bark surfaces from having arm fractures. Mott and her colleagues found that a rubberized impact absorbing surface was safer than bark. Clearly maintenance and depth are important factors in the effectiveness of bark surfaces. Bark surfaces are less expensive than rubberized impact absorbing surfaces to buy but they need much more maintenance.

Equipment

The majority of the playground injuries are equipment related: the surface cannot be considered in isolation from the equipment on it. When exposure is taken into account there are clear differences in the risks to children having injuries on different pieces of equipment. When a child fell from equipment, the probability of receiving an injury on monkey bars was twice that on a climbing frame and seven times that on a swing or slide. Monkey bars are a particular problem for children probably because of the upper body strength and co-ordination needed. Monkey bars add considerably to the risks of children in playgrounds and should not be generally used.

Height

Chalmers et al (1996) in an elegant case-control study from New Zealand clearly showed that the risk of injury was greatly increased at heights of over 1.5 m. The analysis of maximum fall heights by Mott et al (1997) confirms these findings.

Strategies for the future

Children will always have injuries on playgrounds: exploration and testing limits are a natural part of child development. Playgrounds need to remain exciting and challenging to children as they are far safer places to play than alternatives such as the roads. Playground design involves balancing the play value of a playground with safety issues. Safety standards in playgrounds are important and the development of European standards present children with opportunities and threats for their safety. They are at present developed on physical standards only and not on epidemiological data.

A partnership between the Council, the Department of Child Health and the Accident Department can be of value to all. A simple surveillance system in which feedback to the Council can be developed easily (Health Promotion Wales, 1996). This system can react immediately to injuries so that the Council can inspect the site and make changes if necessary. It can also be very useful when developing a playground strategy.

SPORTS INJURIES

All forms of sport and recreation have some risk. The whole ethos of preventing injuries to children during sport and recreation is a difficult one. Clearly, one cannot protect children from all risks in recreational activity, which is important in physical development and the development of personality. On the other hand, one does not want to expose children to unnecessary risk.

Research in sports injury in children is for the most part descriptive. Some studies have added to knowledge about the overall extent of sports injury. Some of these have examined sports injury from the records of the sports clinic treating injuries from organized sports (Watkins and Peabody, 1996). These injuries are characterized by sports in which the participant produces high speed or explosive movements and/or physical contact with other players or apparatus. Others have identified sporting or leisure activities such as rollerblading (Ellis et al, 1995), orienteering (Kujala et al, 1995) and artificial slope skiing (Wyatt and Beatie, 1995) with a view to warning parents and consumers of potential hazards. A third group of studies place sports injury in the context of injuries attending hospital emergency departments. These studies show that sports related injuries are a leading cause of hospital attendance (Nolan and Penny, 1992) and also make a considerable contribution to impairment and disability (Barker et al, 1996).

There has been little research on the risks of various sports, in particular whether rugby or soccer are dangerous for boys. A study in Wales (Hughes et al, 1986) suggested that rugby may cause more injuries than soccer in particular to the upper part of the body. There is also the danger of neck injuries and paraplegia with rugby (McCoy et al, 1984).

Research in sports injuries needs to address the extent of injury in order to set priorities for prevention. Bijur et al (1995) has provided estimates of the extent of the problem of sports injuries for the USA at least. Their study of American 5–14 year olds estimated sports injury to account for 36% of all injury and that 31% of all sports related injury was serious enough for hospitalization, surgical treatment, time off school, or half a day or more in bed. This study provided definitions of sports injury (in terms of international classification of disease (CD) codes). Definitions of sport, recreation and leisure activities are not always clearly stated making comparisons between studies impossible.

An area of sports research that requires further work is the relationship between numbers of injured and the extent of participation in the sporting or recreational activity. In a study of elite young athletes in soccer, gymnastics, tennis and swimming, Baxter-Jones et al (1993) found a rate of less than 1 injury/1000 hours of training. In contrast to the low prevalence of injury found in elite athletes, Gerrard (1993) noted a trend towards high intensity training at a younger age (pre-adolescent) and alerts medical practitioners to be aware of over-enthusiastic parents promoting such training.

Barker et al (1996) have presented an analysis of data from the National Child Development Study, a cohort study of all children born in England, Scotland and Wales in one week in 1958. They studied the risks of disability from injury, and reported that non-life threatening injuries, particularly those to the hand and limb fractures resulting from accidents at work, at home and during sports contribute to the prevalence of permanent injured-related disability in children and young adults. As injury research matures and the scope of the problem is better understood priorities could be the relative merits of addressing high profile fatal injuries, such as those involving motor vehicles, or those low profile emergency department treated injuries that lead to life-long disability or impairment.

There are few recreational activities for children that do not have some risk, nevertheless this risk can be reduced by sensible supervision and other safety measures. Hill and mountain climbing expeditions need careful supervision by experienced guides and teachers if disasters are to be prevented. Rugby teams should be of similar age and ability and referees should pay particular attention to collapsing the scrum.

HORSE ACCIDENTS

Horse riding is a common leisure pursuit, particularly in girls around puberty. Horse riding accidents are one of the few types of accident that are more common in girls than boys (Baker, 1973; Nixon et al, 1981), with the peak incidence in 10–14 year olds. The few deaths each year usually result from severe head injuries. They do not usually reach double figures in England and Wales.

Just under half of horse accidents arise from a fall leading to head injuries, limb fractures and occasionally spinal injuries. Some children get kicked and some are crushed by horses falling on them. Horses also sometimes bite and butt children and tread on their feet.

Many accidents to children on horses are caused by inexperience on the part of the rider particularly when the horse is startled in traffic. Injury during competitions is rare. Good supervision and teaching are important in prevention and horse and rider should be matched. Good head protection is vital in preventing serious head injury. Many traditional riding hats offer little protection for the rider: the new British Standards for protective hats are important for safety.

DROWNING

Drowning continues to be a major cause of death among children in many parts of the world. Particularly high rates have been noted among toddler-age children in parts of the USA, (Wintermute et al, 1991), Australia (Pitt and Balanda, 1991), the UK (Kemp and Sibert, 1991), Japan (Mizuta et al 1993) and Holland (Bierens et al, 1989). In the USA drowning death rates are as high as 1:8000 for boys aged 2–3 years in Los Angeles County (O'Carroll et al, 1988).

Drowning is the third most common cause of accidental death in children in the UK. In 1988 and 1989, 306 children had confirmed submersion incidents: 149 dying and 157 surviving after near drowning (Kemp and Sibert, 1992), 10 of whom sustained severe neurological deficit. The majority were less than 5 years of age. Drowning is an unusual accident and is an infrequent cause of presentation to the accident and emergency department. Many near drowning cases admitted to hospital are seriously ill and have to be admitted to the intensive care unit (Kemp and Sibert, 1991).

Many more boys drown than do girls, which reflects the very different behaviour patterns of boys. There are also very heavy social class gradients, with disadvantaged children more likely to drown. One mode of drowning that does not follow this pattern is death in private swimming pools. The annual incidence in England and Wales of submersion accidents for children under 15 years of age was 1.5/100 000 with a mortality rate of 0.7/100 000. Boys, under 5, had the highest incidence of submersion, 3.6/100 000.

Sites of drowning

Children can drown indoors and outdoors, and in deep or shallow water. Drowning and near drowning in childhood can be divided by the site where the injury takes place. Each site of drowning incident has a definite age range (Kemp and Sibert, 1992) and corresponds to a stage in child development: babies who cannot protect themselves when they fall in bath water, toddlers who wander off and older children who die whilst swimming.

Bath drownings

Bath drownings occur in babies. They can drown in quite shallow water and should not be left unattended. The possibility of non-accidental drowning should be remembered in young children (Nixon and Pearn, 1977; Kemp et al, 1994). Kemp and her colleagues found that accidental bath drownings were confined to children under 2. Bathing in the domestic bathtub is a regular ritual and younger children are at particular risk. Commonly young children are in the bath with older siblings who get out leaving the toddler, with immature developmental skills, to drown in the tub. The domestic bathtub has also been identified as providing particular risk for children with epilepsy. Kemp and Sibert (1993), found 9% of bathtub drownings were related to epilepsy. Diekema et al (1993) reported on 336 submersions and used population based estimates of epilepsy prevalence. They found the relative risk of submersion for children with epilepsy was 47 in the bathtub and 18.7 in the pool. The relative risk of drowning for these children in the bathtub was 96 and 23.4 in the pool. Child Health workers should be prepared to advise parents of children with epilepsy that their children can enjoy the pleasures of water play but that precautions such as not swimming alone or unsupervised and showering rather than bathing in a tub are preferred.

Intentional injury in the bath

The bathtub has been implicated in intentional injury to children. Non-accidental immersion in the bath was identified as an extension of child abuse in 1977 in a total population study of drowning (Nixon and Pearn, 1977). That study reported that about 2% of all drownings and near drownings and 10% of bathtub immersions, could be attributed to this form of child abuse. The data was based on interviews with parents in a research context. Kemp et al (1994) have suggested from a review of 44 bathtub immersions that 10 had inconsistencies and histories suggestive of abuse while Lavelle et al (1995) have estimated that 67% of their retrospective review of bathtub near drownings were suspicious. While these estimates vary dramatically the best advice for emergency department attendants is that child abuse should be considered in the differential diagnosis when a child presents with bathtub immersion and an adequate history and thorough examination be undertaken.

Garden pond drownings

Garden pond drownings occur in toddlers. Children can drown in quite small shallow ponds. The commonest story is of an unsupervised toddler wandering off to a neighbour's house or when visiting friends or relatives. Toddlers can also drown in pails, farm slurry pits, cattle troughs and puddles.

Domestic and private swimming pools

Toddlers and young children are also at a danger when wandering off un-supervised into domestic swimming pools. Unsupervised children may either fall into the pool or crawl under the covers. These drownings are a particular problem in warm affluent countries. Children may also drown in private pools, without supervision, in hotels and holiday camps.

Fencing domestic swimming pools to prevent access by the 0–3 year olds, who are at greatest risk, has been recommended from studies where there has been a high prevalence of pool drownings. Toddler-age children who drown rarely do so after scaling a pool fence. There is one case of a child drowning in an adequately fenced pool from 300 cases in the Brisbane drowning study. In data from New South Wales, Cass et al (1991) reported one case of a child who gained access to a pool by scaling the fence. More commonly the child walks through an unsecured gate or toddles toward an unprotected pool. Whether fencing is promoted through legislative means or education, it should be supported by an educational emphasis on keeping self-closing gates well maintained and shut (Pitt and Balanda, 1991).

Wintermute et al (1991) reported a higher risk of immersion when the occupants had lived in a house with a pool for less than 6 months. Familiarity with the environment and learning to live with hazards is part of growing up. The challenge is to create a safe environment while the vulnerable period passes.

Public pool

Deaths from public pool drownings are a minor problem in the UK following health and safety regulations introduced in 1985, which insist that there is a high level of supervision of children in such pools (Health and Safety Commission 1988). Drownings in public pools are at a level of one per year in the UK: a tribute to the level of supervision (Kemp and Sibert, 1992). Many of the children who are admitted to hospital after nearly drowning in public baths have had effective poolside resuscitation.

Rivers, canal, lakes and sea

Drowning in rivers, canals and lakes is predominantly a problem of older boys who play unsupervised and get into trouble in deep water (Kemp and Sibert, 1992). Many are non-swimmers. These boys correspond to the boys in Australia who drown in creeks. A few children drown at sea in England and Wales, some from falling into docks, some are lost at sea in boating accidents and some drown from the beach.

Differences between countries in which a high drowning incidence has been reported include a different mix of sites. However, the common element seems to be that children drown in water hazards that are close to where they live. In Australia, California and Florida young children predominantly drown in domestic swimming pools, in Holland they drown in canals, in the UK they drown in garden ponds and in Japan they drown in the floor-level home bathtub. Preventive strategies include fencing swimming pools and providing self-closing gates. Where toddlers are concerned the gate is the weak link providing ready access if not secured. The most likely strategy to prevent bathtub drowning on the other hand is education.

Prevention

Most drowning accidents occur with children too young to learn to swim. Preventing bath accidents in babies should be part of the health visitor's programme of education with mothers. It should be emphasized that it is unsafe to leave young children unsupervised in the bath even for short periods. Mothers should also be told about the dangers of drowning in garden ponds and families with young children are well advised to fence or cover these. Much could be done to insist on protecting children from access to these ponds particularly in garden centres. There is evidence that fencing that prevents children from having access to domestic pools with self-closing gates can prevent drowning. Pearn and Nixon (1977) compared drownings from private swimming pools in Brisbane and in Canberra. In Canberra, swimming pools by law had to be fenced but there was no such legal sanction in Brisbane at the time of the study: only one child died in the Australian capital from a swimming pool accident over a 5 year period, compared with 55 in Brisbane. Fencing has been introduced by regulation in Australia, South Africa, New Zealand and parts of the USA. We still await such legislation in the UK.

To be unable to swim probably increases the risk of drowning. Graham and Keating (1978) found evidence that teaching children to swim may have reduced the number of deaths among 5–14 year olds. Certainly, there has been an overall fall in the number of deaths of children from drowning, which has coincided with better swimming training. A number of older children drown whilst swimming unsupervised in rivers, lakes and creeks: this unsupervised swimming should be discouraged but is impossible to prevent. The reduction in drowning in serious public swimming pool incidents with the introduction of health and safety regulations has been most welcome (Kemp and Sibert, 1992). This supervision at the waterside should remain a high priority for local authorities and should be extended to private pools and open water where swimming is common.

Life jackets and buoyancy aids are important in helping to prevent children who use boats and canoes from drowning if they fall overboard. Getting children to wear them is difficult but boat and canoe clubs can insist that their members wear them.

INJURIES AT SCHOOL AND WORK

Injuries at school

The importance of education to children is clearly recognized in the UN Convention on the Rights of the Child (Children's Rights Development Unit, 1994). Injuries occurring to children at school should therefore be a well-researched subject: however the literature is sparse. It seems that the majority of injuries occur during play at breaks and relatively few occur in the class. The same considerations regarding playground design in parks apply to the school with a safe environment for children's play. This is rarely found in schools in the UK. In particular there should be opportunities for constructive play such as is advocated in *Health Promoting Playground* (Health Promotion Wales, 1994)

Injuries at work

Article 32.1 of the UN Convention on the Rights of the Child stresses the right of all children to be protected from work that is 'harmful to the child's health and development'. One of the reasons for this is the increased likelihood of accidents (Children's Rights Development Unit, 1994). A survey in Britain in 1991 (Low Pay Unit and Birmingham City Council Education Department, 1991) indicated that 40% of the population under 16 was working, and of these over a third had had an accident at work in a year. Other information is sparse however. Much more attention should be paid to surveillance and enforcement of regulations throughout the world.

Agricultural injuries

Agriculture is unique in that a significant component of the work force is made up from children under the age of 16, especially at times of peak activity in the farming year. For children, the most significant feature in considering farm related accidents is that the farm is perceived as a place of excitement and adventure. For many, the farm is often also the home, or the place where holidays are taken. The attraction of watching and often helping in farm work, is for many children a valuable and long remembered experience, frequently fostered by parents who wish their children to learn about farming with an eye to their future employment. Nevertheless, it is clear that the farm may be a dangerous environment for children.

Between 1976 and 1988, a total of 167 children in England and Wales were killed as a result of accidents on the farm, representing nearly 25% of all farm related deaths (Royal Society for the Prevention of Accidents, 1988). The problem of farm accidents to children is well recognized in the USA (Rivara, 1985), where approximately 300 children die each year in farm accidents. It has been thought to be of epidemic proportions (Cogbill et al, 1985). In the UK there is a statutory obligation upon employers to report serious injuries and accidents under the Reporting of Injuries, Diseases and Dangerous Occurrences Regulations. Cameron et al (1992) reviewed the problem of farm accidents to children in a 12 month prospective study of child farm accidents in the county of Dyfed, finding one child in 50 living on a farm presents with a farm related accident in a year. None of these non-fatal cases had been reported to RIDDOR.

Cameron et al (1992) also analysed details of all fatal farm accidents to children in Britain over a 4 year period. Tractor related injuries are still the most frequent cause of serious farm related accidents to children. They are well recognized as being likely to cause multiple organ injuries (Rivara, 1987). Legislation to prohibit the driving of tractors by children under the age of 13, and to prohibit the riding of any persons as passengers on either tractors, trailers, or other field implements has been in place for many years but is often ignored. The increasing popularity of farm bikes, particularly three and four wheelers, which may be used off the road without crash helmets, has led to several significant injuries (Cameron et al, 1992). Children are also killed by falls and by objects, particularly tractor wheels, falling on them.

Preventive strategies for agricultural injuries

Educational strategies are an appealing way forward in the prevention of farm injuries but there is little evidence of their effectiveness (Aherin et al, 1992). This is probably because of the isolated nature of many farms and farming communities. A safe community approach is being tried in some places (Ceridigion Farm Safety Group, personal communication).

Clearly safety regulations are important to ensure a safe environment for children. For instance tractor related deaths have fallen (Cameron et al, 1992) since safety regulations have been introduced on design. There are difficulties in enforcement however of the regulations that children should not be allowed to play in, on, or around tractors except under the most scrupulous supervision.

Unless safety regulations are seen to be enforceable and enforced there is likely to be little progress in safety for children on farms. The standard principles of injury prevention with surveillance, adequate regulations and frequent inspection seems to offer the best hope for the future.

REFERENCES

Aherin RA, Murphy DJ & Westby JD (1992) Reducing farm injuries: issues and methods. St Joseph MI: American Society of Agricultural Engineers

Baker HM (1973) Horse play: survey of accidents with horses. *British Medical Journal* 3: 532–534.

Ball D & King K (1991) Playground injuries: a scientific appraisal of popular concerns. *Journal of the Royal Society of Health*. August: 134–137.

Barker M, Power C & Roberts I (1996) Injuries and the risk of disability in teenagers and young adults. *Archives of Disease in Childhood* 75: 156–158.

Baxter-Jones A, Maffulli N & Helms P (1993) Low injury rates in elite athletes: *Archives of Disease in Childhood* 68: 130–132.

Bierens JJ, van der Velde EA, van Berkel M & van Zanten JJ (1989) Submersion cases in the Netherlands. *Annals of Emergency Medicine* 18: 366–373.

Bijur PE, Trumble A, Harel Y, Overpeck MD, Jones D & Scheidt PC (1995) Sports and recreation injuries in US children and adults. *Archives of Pediatric and Adolescent Medicine* 149: 1009–1016.

Cameron D, Bishop C & Sibert JR (1992) Farm accidents in children. *British Medical Journal* 305: 23–25.

Chalmers DJ, Marshall SW, Langley JD et al (1996) Height and surfacing as risk factors in falls from playground equipment: a case-control study. *Injury Prevention* 2: 98–104.

Children's Rights Development Unit (1994) *UK Agenda for Children*. London: Children's Rights Development Unit.

Cogbill TH, Busch HM & Stiers GR (1985) Farm accidents in children. *Pediatrics* 76: 562–566.

Diekema DS, Quan L & Holt VL (1993) Epilepsy as a risk factor for submersion injury in children. *Pediatrics* 91: 612–616.

Ellis JA, Kierulf JC & Klassen TP (1995) Injuries associated with in-line skating from the Canadian hospitals injury reporting and prevention program database. *Canadian Journal of Public Health* 86: 133–136.

Gerrard DF (1993) Overuse injury and growing bones: the young athlete at risk. *British Journal of Sports Medicine* **27**: 14–18.

Health Promotion Wales (1994) *Health Promoting Playground*. Cardiff: Health Promotion Wales.

Health Promotion Wales (1996) *How Safe are Your Playgrounds? Preventing Injuries—Increasing Safety*. Cardiff: Health Promotion Wales.

Heseltine P & Holborn J (1987) *Playgrounds The Planning, Design and Construction of Play Environments*. Mitchell London: 20–27.

Heseltine P, Holborn J & Wenger J (1989) *Playground Management and Safety*. National Playing Fields Association.

Hughes DR, Evans RC & Sibert JR (1986) Sports injuries to children. *British Journal of Accident and Emergency Medicine* **1**: 4–13.

Illingworth C, Brennan P, Jay A, Al-Rawi F & Collick M (1975) 200 injuries caused by playground equipment. *British Medical Journal* **4**: 332–334.

Kemp AM & Sibert JR (1991) Outcome for children who nearly drown: a British Isles study: *British Medical Journal* **302**: 931–933

Kemp AM & Sibert JR (1992) Drowning and near drowning in children in the United Kingdom. Lessons for prevention. *British Medical Journal* **304**: 1143–1146.

Kemp AM & Sibert JR (1993) Epilepsy in childhood and the risk of drowning. *Archives of Disease in Childhood* **68**: 684–685.

Kemp AM, Mott AM & Sibert JR (1994) Accidents and child abuse in bathtub submersions. *Archives of Disease in Childhood* **70**: 435–438.

Kujala UM, Nylund T & Taimela S (1995) Acute injuries in orienteers. *International Journal of Sports Medicine* **16**: 122–125.

Lavelle JM, Shaw KN, Seidl T & Ludwig S (1995) Ten year review of pediatric bathtub near drownings: evaluation for child abuse and neglect. *Annals of Emergency Medicine* **25**: 344–348.

Lewis ML, Naunheim R, Standeven J & Naunheim KS (1993) Quantification of impact attenuation of different playground surfaces under various environmental conditions using a tri-axial accelerometer. *Journal of Trauma* **35**: 932–935.

Low Pay Unit and Birmingham City Council Education Department (1995) *The Hidden Army: Children at Work in the 1990's*. Birmingham: Low Pay Unit and Birmingham City Council.

McCoy GF, Piggott J, Macafee A & Adair IA (1984) Injuries to the cervical spine in schoolboy rugby football. *Journal of Bone and Joint Surgery* **66B**: 500–503.

MacCleary L (1989) *Playgrounds—Leisure Accident Surveillance System (LASS)*. London: Consumer Safety Unit Department of Trade and Industry.

Mizuta R, Fujita H, Osamura T, Kidowaki T & Kiyosawa N (1993) Childhood drownings and near drownings in Japan. *Acta Paediatrica Japonica* **35**: 186–192.

Mott A, Evans R, Rolfe K et al (1994) Patterns of injuries to children on public playgrounds. *Archives of Disease in Childhood* **71**: 328–330.

Mott A, Evans R, Rolfe K et al (1996) *Proceedings of the British Paediatric Association*

Mott A, Evans R, Rolfe K et al (1997) *Proceedings of the Royal College of Paediatrics and Child Health*

Nixon J & Pearn J (1977) Non-accidental immersion in bath-water: another aspect of child abuse. *British Medical Journal* **i**: 271–272.

Nixon J, Pearn J & Wilkey I (1981) Death during play; a study of playground and recreation deaths in children. *British Medical Journal* **282**: 410.

Nixon JW, Kemp AM, Levene S & Sibert JR (1995) Suffocation, choking and strangulation in childhood in England and Wales: epidemiology and prevention. *Archives of Disease in Childhood* **71**: 7–14.

Nolan T & Penny M (1992) Epidemiology of non-intentional injuries in an Australian urban region: results from injury surveillance. *Journal of Paediatrics and Child Health* **28**: 27–35.

O'Carroll PW, Alkon E & Weiss B (1988) Drowning mortality in Los Angeles County 1976 to 1984. *Journal of the American Medical Association* **260**: 380–383.

Pearn JH & Nixon J (1977) Are swimming pools becoming more dangerous? *Medical Journal of Australia* **2**: 702–704.

Pitt WR & Balanda KP (1991) Childhood drowning and near drowning in Brisbane; the contribution of domestic pools. *Medical Journal of Australia* **154**: 661–665.

Rivara FP (1985) Fatal and nonfatal farm injuries to children and adolescents in the United States. *Pediatrics* **76**: 567–573.

Royal Society for the Prevention of Accidents: Birmingham. *Agricultural Safety Listings Report* (1988).

Sacks JJ, Holt KW, Holmgreen P, Colwell LS & Brown JM (1990) Playground hazards in Atlanta Child Care Centers. *American Journal of Public Health* **80:** 986–988.

Watkins J & Peabody P (1996) Sports injuries in children and adolescents treated at a sports injury clinic. *Journal of Sports Medicine and Physical Fitness* **36:** 43–48.

Wintermute GJ, Drake C & Wright M (1991) Immersion events in residential swimming pools. Evidence for an experience effect. *American Journal of Diseases in Children* **145:** 1200–1203.

Wyatt JP & Beattie TF (1995) Paediatric injuries on an artificial ski slope. *Injury* **26:** 87–88.

4

Causes and prevention of road traffic injuries in childhood and adolescence

ELIZABETH M. L. TOWNER MA, BSc, PhD

Senior Lecturer in Community Child Health
Community Child Health, University of Newcastle upon Tyne, Donald Court House, 13 Walker Terrace, Gateshead NE8 1EB, UK

HEATHER WARD BSc, MSc

Principal Research Fellow
Centre for Transport Studies, University College London, Gower Street, London, WC1E 6BT, UK

Within the road environment children can be injured as pedestrians or cyclists when they are moving from place to place, when they are playing, or when they are transported as car occupants. The scale of the problem is enormous around the world and we consider comparative data for different countries. Britain is taken as an example to illustrate some of the patterns of injury, and travel patterns. In order to understand how childhood accidents and injuries can be prevented we need to consider the range of factors that contribute to the accident involvement of children in the road environment. These include immaturity, sex, characteristics of the child, parents and families, adult responsibility for children, risk taking, exposure to injury risk and social deprivation. We consider some of the individual strands and then discuss how these can act in combination. The multifaceted nature of the factors that contribute to injury need to be kept in mind when considering the preventive strategies that are possible and those that have already been demonstrated to be effective. Prevention of such injuries can occur through broad land use and transport policy, education of children and/or their parents and drivers, environmental modification e.g. traffic humps, bicycle helmets and legislation, regulations and enforcement.

Key words: unintentional injury; pedestrian; cyclist; car occupant; injury prevention.

SCALE OF THE PROBLEM

Every day of the year children are injured as they walk, cycle or play in the road environment or when they are being carried as passengers in vehicles. The scale of the problem world-wide is enormous and in the USA alone over 2300 children aged under 15 years were killed on American roads. In Europe about 400 French children were killed and on British roads a further

Baillière's Clinical Paediatrics—
Vol. 5, No. 3, August 1997
ISBN 0–7020–2319–1
0963–6714/97/030373 + 20 $12.00/00

270 died. Rapid motorization in lower income countries has led to greatly increased injuries in the road environment in these countries (Berger and Mohan, 1996).

Figure 1 shows the 1995 fatality rate/100 000 population of children aged 0–14 years for a selection of countries. Figure 2 shows the fatality rate/100 000 child pedestrians for the same group of countries (Department of Transport (DoT) from the International Road Accident Database). The differences between the two figures is interesting. The USA, New Zealand and Portugal have, within this particular and somewhat arbitrary selection of countries, a relatively high road fatality rate for children and for children as pedestrians. Sweden retains its position as being one of the safest countries in the world for children whether they be pedestrians or passengers in vehicles.

However, whilst a child in Britain, or in Japan, appears to be less likely to be killed on the road than a child in France, for example, as pedestrians the fatality rate/100 000 French children is somewhat lower than for British or Japanese children. There are many inter-relating factors that influence these rates and exposure to traffic is an important one. Others are age of the child, gender, socio-economic group, behaviour and the road environment.

In order to illustrate the effects of some of these, Britain will be used as an example but similar factors and patterns will emerge and apply in other countries, albeit with different levels of influence in each country.

According to 1994 population estimates there are about 11.9 million children under the age of 16 in Britain and road accidents account for two

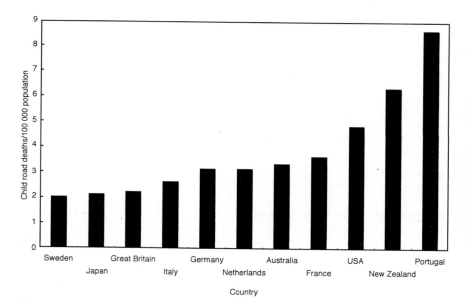

Figure 1. International road deaths/100 000 child population aged 0–14 years in 1995.

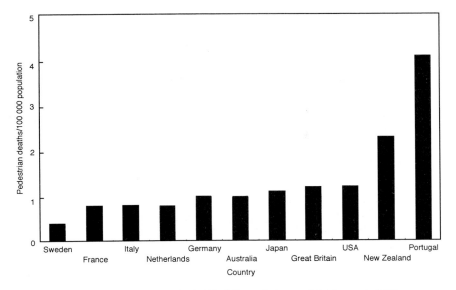

Figure 2. Child pedestrian deaths/100 000 population aged 0–14 years in 1995.

thirds of all accidental deaths of schoolchildren. It has been estimated that 1 in 15 children can expect to be injured in a road accident before their 16th birthday (DoT, 1990). In 1995, 270 children died after being involved in road traffic accidents and a further 6983 sustained serious injuries.

Figure 3 shows trends in the number of child pedestrians killed or seriously injured over the period 1987 to 1995. The number of casualties has fallen for each age group in this period, which is a very positive sign that engineering and education, training and publicity campaigns are having an effect. How much effect is rather difficult to specify because over a period of 20 years or so there have been large changes in the amount of travel by children and the mode by which they travel. According to the National Travel Survey (DoT, 1995) the average mileage walked/child aged 5–10 years has declined by about 9% since 1989/91 and by about 27% since 1975/76. The corresponding reductions in walking for children aged 11–15 years are 17 and 14%. Much of this reduction can be accounted for by changing patterns in car ownership and use.

Although the number of cycles owned/person doubled between 1975/76 and 1992/94, cycle mileage fell substantially. For males aged 5–10 it fell by a third and for females of the same age cycle mileage fell by a half. For the 11–15 age group the reductions were substantially the same for males and females at about 45%.

These changes in travel patterns show through in the casualty statistics and an awareness of these is important when trying to understand changing trends in accident patterns and the relative contributions of different types of interventions.

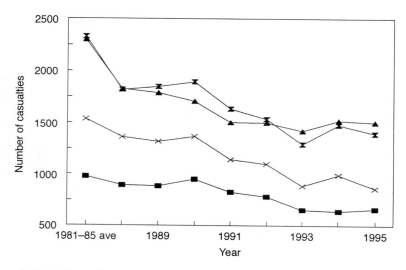

Figure 3. Trends in numbers of child pedestrians killed or seriously injured. Ages of children: —◆—, 0–4 years; —■— 5–7 years, —▲—, 8–11 years; —×—, 12–15 years.

Table 1. Child casualties by age and severity of injury.

Age of child(years)	Severity of injury			All injuries
	Fatal	Serious	Slight	
0–4	54	914	5611	6579
5–7	43	1175	6251	7469
8–11	61	2096	11 123	13 280
12–15	112	2798	13 550	16 460
All children	270	6983	36 535	43 788

Source: Department of Transport (1996).

Table 1 shows child casualties in Britain by age and severity of injury. In the police records of road traffic accidents a fatal injury is defined as death within 30 days, a serious injury encompasses broken bones, severe lacerations or other injuries that require the casualty to be kept in hospital overnight. Slight injuries are classified as, for example, slight cuts and bruising and shock not requiring admission to hospital. The tables of casualties in this section show the numbers that have been reported to the police and entered on the STATS 19 database, which is maintained locally by each police force and nationally by the DoT who publish annually *Road Accidents Great Britain: The Casualty Report*.

It is known that many injuries go unreported, especially where the injury is slight or the child is on a bicycle. One estimate put the level of under-reporting to the police of all child pedestrian casualties at about one quarter (Tunbridge et al, 1988). In a study of pedestrians in Northampton, Ward et al (1994) estimated the under-reporting rate for child pedestrians to be about 20% with boys being less likely to have their injuries reported than girls. To obtain a more accurate picture of the risk of injury it is necessary to consult other sources of casualty information, such as accident and emergency department records, and match to those found in the police records.

About 60% of all deaths and serious injuries are sustained whilst the child is on foot. Child cyclists account for another 17% of these casualties and about the same proportion of the total occur to children as passengers in cars. This illustrates the especial vulnerability of children when out on foot in the road environment.

Patterns of injury are not uniform across the different types of road. Almost all (97%) of child pedestrian injuries occur on roads in built up areas, that is where the speed limit is 40 miles/hour or less, and the pattern for child cyclists is very similar. For occupants of cars and other vehicles about three fifths of the casualties are on built up roads. However, about three fifths of all child occupant fatalities occur on the non-built up roads. Knowledge of these patterns helps target resources on areas where the problem is seen to be greatest.

Within urban areas, a large majority (80%) of younger pedestrians are injured on the residential roads within 1 kilometre of home, with over half being injured within 400 metres of home. As the children grow older they venture further afield and the result of this is that they are injured further from home and an increasing proportion of their injuries (about a third) occur on the main roads that they walk alongside and cross unaccompanied more frequently than do the younger children. For these older children about two thirds of their injuries are within 1 kilometre of home and about 40% within 400 metres.

It is rare to find junctions or short stretches of road in towns and cities where injuries to child pedestrians or cyclists repeatedly occur. The vast majority are scattered over all the roads, especially those in residential areas where children spend much of their time outside the home. The injuries do not occur evenly through the day or through the year. The hours when more child road accidents occur are during the week between 08.00 and 09.00 hours and between 15.00 and 19.00. These periods coincide with the journey to school and home again and with leisure activities after school. About one third of child pedestrian injuries occur on the journey to or from school. Figure 4 shows child casualties/1 000 000 population by hour of the day and by day of the week.

There tends to be a greater number of children injured in the summer months when there is more light and good weather during which they can go out of the home to take part in leisure activities. There are about 4000 casualties each month between May and September compared with about 2800 during the winter months of December to February.

In Britain data on ethnic and social background is not collected by the police when recording road traffic accident data although its collection and use could help focus scarce resources in areas with higher than average casualty rates. Research in Britain indicates that Asian children are over-represented among pedestrian fatalities (e.g. see Lawson, 1990; Lawson and Edwards, 1992). There is also evidence that the number of road traffic

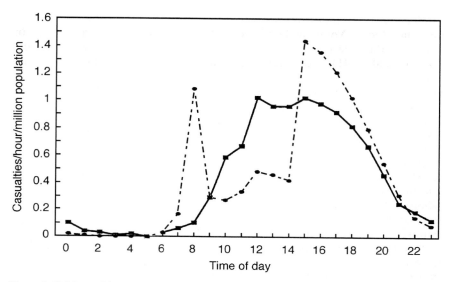

Figure 4. Child casualties (0–15 years) by hour of day: all severities. — · —, Weekday; ——, weekend. Data from DoT (1995).

deaths is related to socio-economic group of the family. These issues are discussed in greater depth in the next section.

BACKGROUND AND CAUSE

In order to understand how childhood accidents and injuries can be prevented we need to consider the range of factors that contribute to the accident involvement of children in the road environment. These include immaturity, sex, characteristics of the child, parents and families, adult responsibility for children, risk taking, exposure to injury risk and social deprivation. We initially consider some of the individual strands and then discuss how these can act in combination.

Factors associated with childhood injuries.

Immaturity

Children are not simply miniature adults. Because of their physical, psychological and behavioural characteristics they are more vulnerable than adults to injuries in the road environment. When the epidemiology of road traffic injuries is examined, the type of accidents children have and where they occur reflects the child's age and stage of development and their exposure to risk at different ages.

When we consider the physical characteristics of children, their size is an important factor. Young pedestrians can be easily masked by parked cars or bushes at the side of the road and are therefore not seen by car drivers (Wilson et al, 1991). Pedestrians are usually struck by the front of a vehicle. Such an impact could result in an adult having a broken leg while a child might have a serious head or neck injury (Wilson et al, 1991).

Psychological factors play an important part. Sandels (1975) in her studies of children in traffic believes that young children are not able to manage the demands of the road environment and that it is 'impossible to fully adapt small children to the road environment'.

Skills to perceive movement and velocity, distance and depth are well developed in adults, but not in children. Children differ from adults in their interpretation of symbols and their ability to orientate the source of a sound (Klein, 1980). What is required in the road environment is the capacity to integrate this information quickly and efficiently. Children's ability to cope in traffic is also limited by attentional abilities (Christie, 1995a). A young child's (aged 2–7 years) tendency to focus on one or two interesting features in the environment can prevent the adequate search for other important features (Phinney et al, reported in Christie, 1995a).

This leads us on to consider that the way in which children behave also differs markedly from adults and makes them more vulnerable to accidents. When children play they do not make time and space calculations. 'Playing toddlers may follow a toy, animal or older child into the street' (Wilson et al, 1991). Older children and young adolescents range more widely than younger children, which may place them in far more dangerous road situations.

Sex

Boys have a higher rate of pedestrian and bicycle injuries but similar rates of car occupant injuries to girls. The increased risk in boys could be due to differences in innate abilities, differences in behaviour or differences in exposure to injury risk. Girls mature earlier and faster than boys but boys at all ages are more co-ordinated than girls in gross motor skills and have faster reaction times (Grossman and Rivara, 1992). Boys and girls behave

Table 2. Numbers of children killed or seriously injured by activity.

Age of child (years)	Numbers of children killed or seriously injured by activity				All killed or seriously injured casualties
	Pedestrians	Cyclists	Car passenger	Other	
0–4	655	19	265	29	968
5–7	857	163	181	17	1218
8–11	1389	432	280	56	2157
12–15	1499	635	573	203	2910
All children	4400	1249	1299	305	7253

Source: Department of Transport (1996).

in different ways in where they play, in risk taking activities and in their range behaviour. These may reflect innate differences in behaviour as well as differences in exposure related to traditional male and female roles in society. Both risk taking activity and exposure to injury risk are discussed later in this chapter.

Characteristics of the child, parents and families

Behavioural factors relating to the characteristics of the child, parents and the family may be associated with higher rates of childhood injury in the road environment. Analysis of the 1958 British Cohort revealed five significant factors: fidgeting, abnormal behaviour and three measures of family disruption or disadvantage, namely crowding, family problems and being removed from the family and placed in the care of the local authority (Pless et al, 1989). Analysis of the 1970 British Cohort looked in particular at the behavioural predictors of injuries (not just road traffic injuries in school-age children) and identified aggression and over-activity in boys to be important factors (Bijur et al, 1988). The results of this study suggest that certain children are less able than others to negotiate their environment safely and this disability is due in part to aspects of their own behaviour (Bijur et al, 1988).

In some circumstances the characteristics of the parent or the family may affect the ability of the parent to provide effective supervision. Thus the incidence of accidents is higher in families headed by a single parent or where children were living with step families (Wadsworth et al, 1983), or where the mother is mentally or physically ill (Backett and Johnston, 1959; Brown and Davison, 1978). The incidence of accidents is also higher in large families (Husband and Hinton, 1972) and where the mother cares for younger siblings, or an elderly relative or works outside the home (Backett and Johnston, 1959).

One important characteristic relating to the child that may be important for the prevention of injuries is that of physical disability. In a study of child pedestrian accidents and road crossing behaviour in Scotland, 14% of children involved in accidents were reported by their parents as having some physical disability (Scottish Development Department, 1989). The most common disabilities were defective eyesight and hearing problems. More research is required in this area, but obviously children with disabilities may be an important target group in injury prevention.

Adult responsibility for children

We need to consider how adults react to children's vulnerability in the road environment. Direct adult supervision of children in the road environment, the responsibilities of drivers and the responsibilities of other adults in society are all facets of this.

Parental supervision has prevented a great number of injuries in the road environment but supervision is not the panacea, for as Wilson et al (1991) point out parents would need, 'encyclopaedic knowledge, unlimited resources, unyielding vigilance, and constant control of the child's behaviour' to keep their children entirely free from danger. Certain characteristics of the mother/parent and family can impair the ability of the parent to provide effective supervision at all times: if the mother is mentally or physically ill, large families, lone parents etc, and these have already been discussed. Parents can be unrealistic about the age at which children can be expected to cope with traffic (Sandels, 1975). Sharples et al (1990) in a study of children who had died as a result of a head injury in the Northern Region of England found that 53% were playing at the time. Nearly half of these were under 7 years old and only one child was under adult supervision at the time. Many were supervised by older siblings or childhood friends, but these children are also very young. Many of these children lived in overcrowded neighbourhoods that lacked safe places where children could play.

Some children can become involved in pedestrian accidents despite adult supervision. Sandels describes circumstances where children escape from adult supervision suddenly and become involved in an accident (Sandels, 1975). van der Molen et al (1983) observed the crossing behaviour of children accompanied by their parents and found that parents often did not provide much instruction or act as good role models to their children. This provides some evidence that some supervision skills can be enhanced by teaching, but supervision in an inherently dangerous environment may not always be possible, and protection needs also to be built into the environment and into the way society operates (Wilson et al, 1991).

Recognizing and compensating for these developmental handicaps that put child pedestrians at increased risk is important not just for parents but also for adults as vehicle drivers. Drivers are often ill prepared for the unpredictable behaviour of child pedestrians and the presence of children by the roadside does not affect the drivers' speed or position in the road (Thompson et al, 1985). Howarth and Gunn (1982) and Preston (1990) argue that drivers should be more responsible in law for accidents with child pedestrians. Children can be adversely affected by the actions of adult drunk drivers. In the USA about 15% of the traffic related mortality and 10% of the morbidity in children under the age of 15 has been estimated to result from alcohol-related crashes (Margolis et al, 1986).

When considering the wider responsibility of adults in society to the protection of children in the road environment, Hillman et al (1990) argue that 'children's issues in transport planning have been marginalized by policies accommodating the growth in the demand for motor transport'. This has resulted in 'the loss of the street as accessible communal play space' (Hillman et al, 1990). They raise the importance of cultural differences in community supervision of children in the road environment in Germany and Britain (Hillman et al, 1990).

Risk taking

Risk taking behaviour appears to play a major role in the increased rate of injuries amongst adolescents, particularly in older adolescents when they start driving (Grossman and Rivara, 1992). Risk taking behaviour may allow the adolescent to express a sense of control of his or her life, opposition to authority and allow adolescents to be accepted in a peer group (Grossman and Rivara, 1992). Thuen et al (1992) found that risk seeking and low level of safety seeking amongst adolescents were part of a health compromising lifestyle: unhealthy food habits, smoking and alcohol consumption. Safety seeking behaviour included the use of bicycle helmets, clothing reflectors and seat belts, and risk-seeking behaviour included, 'cycling downhill as fast as you can'. A low level of the former and high level of the latter seemed to be embedded in a somewhat deviant or rule-compromising behaviour pattern (Thuen, 1994).

Exposure to injury risk

The amount of time a child spends in the road environment as a pedestrian, a cyclist or car occupant, the type of activities, they do, such as the number of roads they cross, whether they wear seatbelts in cars or protective equipment such as bicycle helmets may have an effect on the nature and severity of injuries they experience in the road environment.

Researchers in Nottingham attempted to measure children's exposure to risk as pedestrians using a variety of interview and observational methods (Routledge et al, 1974). Most child pedestrian accidents occur at road junctions, suggesting that it might be more dangerous to cross the road at a junction than elsewhere. However, when children were observed crossing roads it was possible to take exposure to risk into account and it was found that a child had a higher risk of an accident at a straight road crossing place rather than at a junction (Howarth and Repetto-Wright, 1978). Such information on exposure will help in targeting messages more accurately.

Tight (1987) investigated the accident involvement and exposure to risk for children as pedestrians on urban roads in five towns in England. He found that girls were accompanied more than boys, that accompaniment decreased with age and number of streets crossed increased with age. Children in the North had higher levels of street play than those in the South of England. The accident risk of crossing a main road was 10 times that of crossing a side road, and of crossing a main road not using the crossing facility was three times the risk of crossing such a road using a crossing facility (Tight, 1987). In a study of exposure to risk of 11–14 year old pedestrians and cyclists in Newcastle, poorer children were found to be more exposed to risks than more affluent children (Towner et al, 1994).

Ward and her colleagues conducted a study of over 1000 people in Northampton that looked at the relative risk of pedestrians of different age and gender walking in different types of road environment (Ward et al, 1994). This study related exposure to injuries that took place and found that 'boys and girls aged 5–9 had similar casualty rates per kilometre walked, but boys were 1½ times more likely to be injured when crossing the road. Girls aged 10–15 appeared to be less able than boys of the same age either to walk along side or to cross the road safely. Indeed girls of this age have the highest casualty risk of any age group for both kilometre walked along

side traffic and per roads crossed, (Ward et al, 1994). Using exposure data
in conjunction with injury event data we have a clearer picture to allow us
to target preventive activities to particular target groups or to particular
circumstances or to promote particular messages. A study is currently
underway (funded by the Department of Transport), which investigates
exposure of children to traffic in different European countries.

Many of the exposure studies have concentrated on children as
pedestrians rather than children using streets for play. Christie (1995a)
considers that the measurements for exposure while playing out on the
street pose a methodological problem. Play is dynamic and unstructured
and often unsupervised and parents' response to their children's where-
abouts while playing is likely to underestimate their exposure. All this
makes it difficult to track and codify recreational use of the road environment accurately (Christie, 1995a).

Socio-economic factors

Children from lower income families are much more likely to be injured in
the road environment than those from higher income families. In Britain
there are four times as many pedestrian deaths in children in social class V
than in social class I (OPCS, 1988) and child pedestrian casualty rates are
highest in deprived inner city areas (King et al, 1987; Preston, 1992). This
association has also been found in the USA (Mueller et al, 1990) and
Canada (Pless and Arsenault, 1987). Roberts and his colleagues in New
Zealand found that risk of child pedestrians was strongly associated with
traffic volumes, with risks at the busiest sites 14 times greater than in less
busy sites (Roberts et al, 1995). In these studies, children from lower
income levels lived in areas with busier streets, multi-family dwellings
without play areas and where there was greater exposure to vehicle traffic.

Socio-economic deprivation has also been linked to the dispro-
portionately high incidence of road traffic accidents involving children
from ethnic minorities. Lawson and Edwards (1991) have shown in
Birmingham, England that Asian children under 9 years are twice as likely
to be injured as their non-Asian counterparts. This could partly be
explained by where children live (inner city areas) and where there is more
traffic. A similar finding is reported from Paris by Tursz et al (1991) for
immigrant children. The immigrant children were more likely to live in
homes that had less space to play and children were forced to play out in
the streets.

Many of the factors already discussed in this chapter come together in
considering why child pedestrian casualty rates vary significantly with
socio-economic group. Christie (1995b) conducted a case control study
using home interviews with 152 children injured as pedestrians and 484
school children matched as controls. The problem of child pedestrian
injuries was found to be multi-faceted. There are a great number of different factors that influence the accident involvement of child pedestrians,
some of which are highly correlated with socio-economic group. The
demographic, social and economic factors found to be important are age,

sex and physical capabilities (particularly hearing level) of the child; the marital status, ethnic origin, risk and responsibility scores of the parent/carer and the number of children in the family that the parent has to care for. The amount of street play, level of adult accompaniment and the extent of extra mural activity were important factors relating to exposure. Features of the environment that proved significant were the low levels of on-street parking (this finding was difficult to interpret, but it could be that there is an interaction between vehicle access and the level of parking restriction) and the age of housing. Pre-1914 housing developments featured strongly as a high risk environment (Christie, 1995b).

PREVENTION OF CHILDHOOD INJURY IN THE ROAD ENVIRONMENT

Prevention of childhood injuries in the road environment can occur through broad policy change, through education, environmental modification and legislation and enforcement. The multi-faceted nature of the factors that contribute to injury need to be kept in mind when considering the preventive strategies that are possible and those that have already been demonstrated to be effective. The section below draws widely on a systematic review of the world literature (Dowswell et al, 1996; Towner et al, 1996).

Broad land use and transport policy

Land use and transport policy have a potentially important part to play in reducing childhood injuries on the roads. There is however, limited evidence from the evaluated studies in this field but we are able to make inferences from other forms of evidence. Removal of subsidies from public transport in London led to increased traffic volumes and increased road casualties (Allsop and Turner, 1986). A greater emphasis on public rather than private transport could potentially reduce road traffic accidents. Different types of housing area generate different child casualty rates. King et al (1987) found high child accident casualties in streets of Victorian terrace houses with little or no gardens, few garages and much on-street parking compared with post-war housing estates. They suggest that road safety should be included in objectives of environmental improvement with the density of child accidents in inner city areas being one of the criteria used in the selection of development areas. Policies on land use can influence injury rates. Preston (1972) showed that during the 1970s in England an increase in school size was associated with increased journey times on school journeys and a corresponding increase in child casualties.

Developers and planners laying out new communities have an ideal opportunity to ensure child pedestrian and cyclist safety. Examples include 'separating pedestrians from traffic and ensuring walking routes to schools and parks that do not force children to cross major roads' (Wilson et al,

1991). Child road safety issues need to be higher on the agenda of policy makers and planners and there is a need for further research to measure the impact of policy changes on child road injury patterns (Towner et al, 1996).

Local changes in the road environment

There is good evidence that local changes in the road environment by area wide engineering measures have reduced injury rates to child pedestrians and child cyclists. A number of studies have been conducted in Denmark, Germany, the Netherlands and Britain (Towner et al, 1996). One study in the Netherlands used data over a 15 year period to compare the effectiveness of three different models of road safety measures: (a) very simple measures to exclude through traffic from residential areas; (b) more extensive measures to exclude most local traffic and to limit the speed of traffic; (c) the complete reconstruction of the road environment to give pedestrians priority (Janssen, 1991). The second of these interventions, the intermediate treatment proved to be the most successful and reduced injuries by up to 25% (Janssen, 1991).

In England the Urban Safety Project was evaluated in five towns: Reading, Nelson, Sheffield, Bradford and Bristol, with each town having an intervention and control area with similar road accident rates (Lynam et al, 1988). Interventions were introduced that redistributed traffic and improved the safety of individual stretches of road. For example sheltered parking, right hand turning bays and road closures. The road traffic injuries occurring over a 7 year period were measured and an overall reduction in accidents of 13% occurred (Mackie et al, 1990). There were considerable variation between the towns, but in one town (Sheffield) there were significant reductions amongst child cyclists and pedestrians (Ward et al, 1989). Lessons learnt in these demonstration projects have been incorporated into local authority traffic safety guidelines (Institute of Highways and Transportation, 1990). A Safer City initiative is currently underway in Gloucester, which is using a multi-agency approach.

Education aimed at the driver

In the previous section we discussed the child's vulnerability in the road environment and the lack of appreciation of this vulnerability by the driver. There is a strong link between vehicle speed and the severity of injury sustained by pedestrians after collision (Kimber, 1990). Campaigns aimed at reducing speed have considerable potential to save children's lives and reduce the severity of their injuries in the road environment.

A campaign in Canada has acknowledged the role of both drivers and pedestrians in road safety rather than focusing solely on the child (Malenfant and Van Houten, 1989). The multi-faceted approach used road engineering measures, school based education and enforcement in its programme to increase the safety of pedestrians at crossing facilities. The programme produced increases in the percentages of motorists yielding the right of way to pedestrians (Malenfant and Van Houten, 1989).

Education aimed at the child and their carers

Traffic clubs have been organized in a number of countries. The Tufty Club developed in the UK has been used in schools and by the parents of pre-school children (Firth, 1973). Results of the evaluation of the Tufty Club have been mixed with knowledge gains reported in one study but not in another (Antaki et al, 1986; Firth, 1973). In Norway children's traffic clubs were developed that emphasized practical instruction and training by parents. Schioldborg (1976) reported lower casualty rates for traffic club members in Norway, but these could probably be explained by selective club membership.

Similar traffic clubs have been introduced in other European countries. In the UK a pilot version of the traffic club, the Streetwise Kids Club was introduced in London but membership was low, particularly in low socio-economic groups (Downing, 1987). A larger scale club, the Eastern Region Traffic Club showed increased membership with all social groups repre-sented. An early evaluation of this club showed an effect on children's behaviour and the number of children running on ahead of parents when out walking was reduced, but there was no effect on children playing un-supervised in the streets or riding bicycles unsupervised (West et al, 1993). Recent evidence of casualty reductions as a result of the Club relate to children emerging from behind parked vehicles (Bryan-Brown, 1993). An evaluation of a traffic club in Sweden found that club members reported more accidents among club members than in controls but this finding could be explained by reporting bias in the intervention group (Gregersen and Nolen, 1994).

Inclusion of parents as well as their children in pedestrian skills training was found to improve behaviour in studies conducted in the USA (Rivara et al, 1991) and the Netherlands (van der Molen et al, 1983). In the latter programme, parents subsequently set better examples to children they accompanied and gave more verbal instructions (van der Molen et al, 1983). Other trials suggest that teaching children road crossing skills can change reported behaviour and instruction in the classroom can be as effective as at the roadside (van Schagen, 1988; Ampofo-Boateng et al, 1993).

Based on experimental studies, the 'Let's Decide Walk Wise' pedestrian training programme for 5–8 year olds has been developed for schools (Harland and Tucker, 1995). This programme includes a curriculum component backed up with practical training in the local environment and work using a table top model. Children in the participating schools showed greater improvements in crossing behaviour than those in controls (Harland and Tucker, 1995), a similar finding to programmes in Australia (Penna, 1994). In the Netherlands both theoretical and practical training of young cyclists to behave correctly at traffic intersections had little effect (van Schagen and Brookhuis, 1994). Observations of children in traffic suggested that children applied informal rather than formal rules when dealing with traffic and these informal rules needed to be the starting point for training activities (van Schagen and Brookhuis, 1994).

Cycle helmets

In an analogous argument to targeting child pedestrians and developing skills programmes, the strategy of promoting cycle helmet wearing can be considered to divert attention from a strategy based on tackling the source of accidents in which cyclists are injured (Hillman, 1993). Nevertheless there is good evidence that most cyclists killed on the roads sustain head injuries (Mills, 1989) and that cycle helmets offer some protection from head injuries, although helmets will not protect a cyclist in a high velocity impact (Dorsch et al, 1987). There is some debate about the relative protective effects of cycle helmets (Thompson et al, 1989; Spaite et al, 1991; Thomas et al, 1994).

An early campaign to promote cycle helmet wearing took place in Seattle (Bergman et al, 1990). The campaign used a wide range of organizations and a range of educational methods. It was highly focused in terms of age group and message and it addressed the issue of the cost of helmets by subsidies. Observed helmet wearing rates increased from 5 to 14% in the target population (Bergman et al, 1990). There is some evidence that increased cycle helmet wearing is achieved in young children rather than teenagers (Finch et al, 1993) and in high income areas (Parkin et al, 1993). The passage of a bicycle helmet law in one country in the USA enabled a comparison to be made of legislative and educational approaches. Legislation combined with education was more effective than education alone in encouraging the use of cycle helmets (Dannenberg et al, 1993).

One major evaluation of the effects of community wide programmes and legislation showed a significant reduction in the rate and severity of casualties. In 1990, following a decade of educational campaigns, Victoria introduced the first legislation in the world requiring cyclists to wear helmets (Leicester et al, 1991; Cameron et al, 1992). Helmet wearing rates increased from 31% before to 75% in the year following legislation and this was associated with a 48% reduction in head injury admission on deaths between 1989/90 and 1990/91 and a reduction of 70% over the 2 year period 1989/90 to 1991/92 (Cameron et al, 1994). Some of the reduction can be explained by a decrease in cycling, particularly in some groups such as teenagers. The reduction in non-head injuries was 23% in the first year and 28% over the first 2 years. At last half the head injury reductions is thus likely to be due to increased wearing of helmets (Cameron et al, 1994; McDermott, 1995).

Protection of car passengers

A high proportion of deaths and severe injuries to motor vehicle occupants can be prevented by the use of appropriate restraints (Agran et al, 1987; Christian and Bullimore, 1989; Wilson et al, 1991). A number of studies have examined the effect of legislation on the use of child restraints and most have reported increases in restraint use (Williams and Wells, 1981) and some reductions in injuries and deaths (Decker et al, 1984). As with bicycle helmet legislation, legislation for child safety restraints needs to be preceded by educational campaigns. In the USA however, legislation has not resulted in universal compliance and restraint usage rates of 40–50% are reported. Seekins et al (1988) compared usage rates in different states and found that compliance was higher in states with greater enforcement. In Britain, an evaluation of the 1983 legislation of front seat belt restraints, found that there was a marked reduction in children aged 11–14 travelling in the front seat (Lowne et al, 1984).

For infants and young children loan schemes and educational campaigns have met with some success in promoting correct restraint use (Reisinger and Williams, 1978; Goodson et al, 1985). Particularly in low income communities gains were often modest (Berger et al, 1984). A community-based injury prevention programme in Massachusetts USA, the Statewide Child Injury Prevention Program (SCIPP) targeted five specific programmes in pre-school children. But the only area where there was a significant reduction in injuries was for motor vehicle passengers (Guyer et al, 1989).

Several campaigns encouraging older children to 'buckle up' have had mixed results. The USA 'Bucklebear' programme used in day-care centres and nursery schools was successful in increasing children's use of safety seats or seat belts (Cheng, et al, 1985). A school based campaign in primary school children used rewards to increase seat belt-use (Roberts and Fanurik, 1986): this had some effect on the children as well as other car occupants. Another study attempted to increase car restraint use through changes to the culture at the child care centres the children attended (Stuy et al 1993).

Conclusion

There is evidence from Australia that the road fatality rate (for all ages) has been reduced from 30/100 000 in 1970 to 11.2/100 000 in 1992, despite the amount of traffic doubling. This has been achieved through 'a strategic mix of legislation and enforcement, education and behaviour change, and engineering and technology approaches', (reported in Commonwealth Department of Human Services and Health, 1994). Support from national and regional government is needed to stimulate large scale initiatives. But work at a local level involving local people is also essential.

REFERENCES

Agran PF, Dunkle DE & Winn DG (1987) Effects of legislation on motor vehicle injuries to children. *American Journal of Diseases of Children* **141:** 959–964.

Allsop RE & Turner ED (1986) Road casualties and public transport fares in London. *Accident Analysis and Prevention* **18:** 147–156.

Ampofo-Boateng K, Thomson JA, Grieve R, et al (1993) A developmental and training study of children's ability to find safe routes to cross the road. *British Journal of Developmental Psychology* **11:** 31–45.

Antaki C, Morris PE & Flude BM (1986) The effectiveness of the *'Tufty Club'* in road safety education. *British Journal of Educational Psychology* **56:** 363–365.

Backett EM & Johnston AM (1959) Social patterns of road accidents to children. Some characteristics of vulnerable families. *British Medical Journal* **1:** 409–413.

Berger LR & Mohan D (1996) *Injury Control A Global View.* Delhi: Oxford University Press.

Berger LR, Saunders S, Armitage K, et al (1984) Promoting the use of car safety devices for infants: an intensive health education approach. *Pediatrics* **74:** 16–19.

Bergman A, Rivara F, Richards D et al (1990) The Seattle children's bicycle helmet campaign. *American Journal of Diseases of Children* **144:** 727–731.

Bijur P, Golding J, Haslum M et al (1988) Behavioural predictors of injury in school-age children. *American Journal of Diseases of Children* **142:** 1307–1312.

Brown G & Davison S (1978) Social class, psychiatric disorder of mother, and accidents to children. *Lancet* **i** 378–380.

Bryan-Brown K (1993) *The effectiveness of the General Accident Eastern Region Children's Traffic Club.* Project Report no 99. Crowthorne: Transport Research Laboratory.

Cameron M, Heiman L & Neiger D (1992) *Evaluation of the Bicycle Helmet Wearing Law in Victoria During its First 12 Months.* Victoria, Australia: Monash University Accident Research Centre (MUARC).

Cameron M, Vulcan A, Finch C et al (1994) Mandatory bicycle helmet use following a decade of helmet promotion in Victoria, Australia—An evaluation. *Accident Analysis and Prevention* **26 26:** 325–337.

Cheng A, Dillman A, Leonard E et al (1985) Teaching car passenger safety to preschool children. *Pediatrics* **76:** 425–428.

Christian M & Bullimore D (1989) Reduction in accident severity in rear seat passengers using restraints. *Injury* **20:** 262–264.

*Christie N (1995a) *Social, Economic and Environmental Factors in Child Pedestrian Accidents: A Research Review.* Project Report no. 116. Crowthorne: Transport Research Laboratory.

*Christie N (1995b) *The High Risk Child Pedestrian: Socio-economic and Environmental Factors in their Accidents.* Project Report no. 117. Crowthorne: Transport Research Laboratory.

Commonwealth Department of Human Services and Health (1994) *Better Health Outcomes for Australians.* Canberra: Commonwealth of Australia Publishing Service.

Dannenberg A, Gielen A, Beilenson P et al (1993) Bicycle helmet laws and educational campaigns: an evaluation of strategies to increase children's helmet use. *American Journal of Public Health* **83:** 667–674.

Decker M, Dewey M, Hutcheson R et al (1984) The use and efficacy of child restraint devices. The Tennessee experience, 1982 and 1983. *Journal of the American Medical Association* **252:** 2571–2575.

Dorsch M, Woodward A & Somers R (1987) Do bicycle safety helmets reduce the severity of head injuries in real crashes? *Accident Analysis and Prevention* **19:** 183–190.

*DoT (Department of Transport) (1990) *Children and Roads: A Safer Way. Government Proposals for Reducing the Number of Child Casualties on our Roads.* London: Department of Transport.

DoT (Department of Transport) (1995) *National Travel Survey 1992/94. Transport Statistics Report.* London: HMSO.

DoT (Department of Transport) (1996) *Road Accidents Great Britain 1995. The Casualty Report.* London: HMSO.

Downing C (1987) Evaluation of the Impact and Penetration of a Children's Traffic Club. Paper presented at the 2nd International Conference on Road Safety, Groningen, 1987.

Dowswell T, Towner E, Simpson G et al (1996) Preventing childhood unintentional injuries—what works? A literature review. *Injury Prevention* **2:** 140–149.

Finch C, Newstead S, Cameron M et al (1993) Head injury reduction in Victoria 2 years after introduction of mandatory bicycle helmet use (Report no. 51). Victoria, Australia: Monash University Accident Research Centre (MUARC).

Firth D (1973) *The Road Safety Aspects of the Tufty Club* (Dept Env Report No LR604) Crowthorne: Department of Transport & Road Research Laboratory.

Goodson J, Buller C & Goodson W (1985) Prenatal child safety education. *Obstetrics and Gynaecology* **65:** 312–315.

Gregersen NP & Nolen S (1994) Children's road safety and the strategy of voluntary traffic safety clubs. *Accident Analysis and Prevention* **26:** 463–470.

Grossman D & Rivara F (1992) Injury control in childhood. *Pediatric Clinics of North America* **39:** 471–485.

Guyer B, Gallagher S, Chang B et al (1989) Prevention of childhood injuries: evaluation of the Statewide Childhood Injury Prevention Program (SCIPP). *American Journal of Public Health* **79:** 1521–1527.

Harland G & Tucker S (1995) 'Let's Decide Walk Wise'—the Development and Testing of a Pedestrian Training Resource. Crowthorne: Transport Research Laboratory.

Hillman M (1993) *Cycle Helmets: The Case For and Against.* London: Policy Studies Institute.

*Hillman M, Adams J & Whitelegg J (1990) *One False Move: A Study of Children's Independent Mobility.* London: Policy Studies Institute.

Howarth C & Gunn M (1982) Pedestrian safety and the law. In Chapman A, Wade F & Foot H (eds) *Pedestrian Accidents,* pp. 265–289. Chichester: John Wiley & Sons.

Howarth C & Repetto-Wright R (1978) The Measurement of Risk and the Attribution of Responsibility for Child Pedestrian Accidents. *Safety Education* **144:** 10–14.

Husband P & Hinton P (1972) Families of children with repeated accidents to children. *Archives of Disease in Childhood* **47:** 396–400.

Institute of Highways and Transportation (1993) *Guidelines for Urban Safety Management.* London: Institute of Highways and Transportation.

Janssen STMC (1991) Road safety in urban districts: final results of accident studies in the Dutch demonstration projects of the 1970s. *Traffic Engineering and Control* (June 1991): 292–296.

Kimber R (1990) Appropriate speeds for different road conditions. In *Parliamentary Advisory Council for Transport Safety. Speed Accidents and Injury, Reducing the Risks.* London: PACTS

King D, Lawson S, Proctor S et al (1987) Child pedestrian accidents in inner areas: patterns and treatment. Paper presented at the PTRC Summer Annual Meeting, University of Bath.

Klein D (1980) Societal influences on childhood accidents. *Accident Analysis and Prevention* **12:** 275–281.

Lawson S (1990) *Accidents to Young Pedestrians: Distribution, Circumstances, Consequences and Scope for Countermeasures.* Basingstoke: AA Foundation for Road Safety Research and Birmingham City Council.

Lawson SD & Edwards PJ (1991) The involvement of ethnic minorities in road accidents: data from three studies of young pedestrian casualties. *Traffic Engineering and Control* (January): 12–19.

Leicester P Nassam F & Wise A (1991) *The Introduction of Compulsory Bicycle Helmet Wearing in Victoria.* Vic. Roads Report, GR 91–4. Victoria, Australia: Victoria Roads.

Lowne R, Roberts A, Roy P et al (1984) *The Effect of the UK Seat Belt Legislation on Restraint Usage by Children.* Technical Paper Series 840526: Society of Automotive Engineers (SAE).

Lynam D, Mackie A & Davies C (1988) *Urban Safety Project. 1. Design and Implementation of Schemes.* Research Report no. 153 Department of Transport, Transport and Road Research Laboratory.

McDermott FT (1995) Bicyclist head injury prevention by helmets and mandatory wearing legislation in Victoria, Australia. *Annals of the Royal College of Surgeons of England* **77:** 38–44.

*Mackie A, Ward H & Walker R (1990) *Urban Safety Project. 3. Overall Evaluation of Area Wide Schemes.* Research Report no. 263. Crowthorne: Transport and Road Research Laboratory.

Malenfant L & Van Houten R (1989) Increasing the percentage of drivers yielding to pedestrians in three Canadian cities with a multifaceted safety program. *Health Education Research* **5:** 275–279.

Margolis L, Kotch J & Lacy J (1986) Children in alcohol related motor vehicle crashes. *Pediatrics* **77:** 870–872.

Mills P (1989) Pedal cycle accidents—a hospital based study. Research Report no. 220. Crowthorne: Department of Transport & Road Research Laboratory.

van der Molen H, van den Herik J & van der Klaauw C (1983) Pedestrian behaviour of children and accompanying parents during school journeys: an evaluation of a training programme. *British Journal of Educational Psychology* **53:** 152–168.

Mueller B, Rivara F, Lii & S-M et al (1990) Environmental factors and the risk for childhood pedestrian-motor vehicle collision occurrence. *American Journal of Epidemiology* **132:** 550–560.

OPCS (Office of Population Censuses and Surveys) (1988) *Occupational Mortality: Childhood Supplement. Registrar General's Decennial Supplement for England and Wales, 1979–80, 1982–83, Vol. 8.* London: HMSO.

Parkin P, Spence L, Hu & X et al (1993) Evaluation of a promotional strategy to increase bicycle helmet use by children. *Pediatrics* **91:** 772–777.

Penna C (1994) 'Streets ahead' evaluation Victoria Roads Report (GR94-13). Victoria, Australia, Victoria Roads.

Pless I & Arsenault L (1987) The role of health education in the prevention of injuries to children. *Journal of Social Issues* **43:** 87–103.

Pless I, Peckham C & Power C (1989) Predicting traffic injuries in childhood: a cohort analysis. *Journal of Pediatrics* **115:** 932–938.

Preston B (1972) Statistical analysis of child pedestrian accidents in Manchester and Salford. *Accident Analysis and Prevention* **4:** 323–332.

Preston B (1990) Home zones—child's play for inner cities. *Town and Country Planning* (April): 116–117.

Preston B (1992) *Cutting Pedestrian Casualties: Cost-Effective Ways to Make Walking Safer.* London: Transport 2000.

Reisinger K & Williams A (1978) Evaluation of programs designed to increase the protection of infants in cars. *Pediatrics* **62:** 280–287.

Rivara FP, Booth CL, Bergman AB et al (1991) Prevention of pedestrian injuries to children: effectiveness of a school training program. *Pediatrics* **88:** 770–775.

Roberts I, Norton R, Jackson R et al (1995) Effect of environmental factors on risk of injury of child pedestrians by motor vehicles: a case-control study. *British Medical Journal* **310:** 91–94.

Roberts M & Fanurik D (1986) Rewarding elementary school children for their use of safety belts. *Health Psychology* **5:** 185–196.

Routledge D, Repetto-Wright R & Howarth CI (1974) Children's exposure to risk as pedestrians. *Ergonomics* **17:** 623–638.

*Sandels S (1975) *Children in Traffic*, revised edn. Surrey: Elek Books Ltd.

van Schagen I (1988) Training children to make safe crossing decisions. In Rothengatter J & de Bruin R (eds) *Road User Behaviour: Theory and Research*, pp. 482–489. Maastricht: van Gorcum.

van Schagen I & Brookhuis K (1994) Training young cyclists to cope with dynamic traffic situations. *Accident Analysis and Prevention* **26:** 223–230.

Schioldborg P (1976) Children, traffic and traffic training: analysis of the children's traffic club. *The Voice of the Pedestrian* **6.**

Scottish Development Department (1989) *Must Do Better. A Study of Child Pedestrian Accidents and Road Crossing Behaviour in Scotland.* Edingburgh: Scotish Office. Consultants' report to Scottish Development Department by MVA Consultancy.

Seekins T, Fawcett S, Cohen S et al (1988) Experimental evaluation of public policy: the case of state legislation for child passenger safety. *Journal of Applied Behavior Analysis* **21:** 233–243.

Sharples P, Storey A, Aynsley-Green A et al (1990) Causes of fatal childhood accidents involving head injury in Northern region, 1979–86. *British Medical Journal* **301:** 1193–1197.

Spaite D, Murphy M, Criss E et al (1991) A prospective analysis of injury severity among helmeted and nonhelmeted bicyclists involved in collisions with motor vehicles. *Journal of Trauma* **31:** 1510–1516.

Stuy M, Green M & Doll J (1993) Child care centers: a community resource for injury prevention. *Journal of Developmental and Behavioral Pediatrics* **14:** 224–229.

Thomas S, Acton C, Nixon J et al (1994) Effectiveness of bicycle helmets in preventing head injury in children: case control study. *British Medical Journal* **308:** 173–176.

Thompson J, Fraser E & Howarth C (1985) Driver behaviour in the presence of child and adult pedestrians. *Ergonomics* **28:** 1469–1474.

Thompson R, Rivara F & Thompson D (1989) A case-control study of the effectiveness of bicycle safety helmets. *New England Journal of Medicine* **320:** 1361–1367.

Thuen F (1994) Injury-related behaviours and sensation seeking: an empirical study of a group of 14 year old Norweigan school children. *Health Education Research* **9:** 465–472.

Thuen F, Klepp KI & Wold B, (1992) Risk-taking and safety-seeking behaviours: a study of health-related behaviours among Norwegian school children. *Health Education Research* **7:** 269–276.

Towner E, Jarvis S, Walsh S et al (1994) Measuring exposure to injury risk in schoolchildren aged 11–14. *British Medical Journal* **308:** 449–452.

*Towner E, Dowswell T, Simpson G et al (1996) *Health Promotion in childhood and Young Adolescence for the Prevention of Unintentional Injuries*, vol. 1, 1st edn. London: Health Education Authority.

Tunbridge RJ, Everest JT, Wild BR & Johnstone RA (1988) *An In-depth Study of Road Accident Casualties and Their Injury Patterns.* Report RR 136-7. Crowthorne: Transport & Road Research Laboratory.

Tursz A, Crost M & Lavaud J (1991) Childhood Traffic Injuries in France: From Epidemiology to Preventative Measures. Paper presented at the Proceedings of the International Conference on Traffic Safety, New Delhi. January, 1991, pp. 195–198. New Delhi: Macmillian India.

Wadsworth J, Burnell I, Taylor B et al (1983) Family type and accidents in preschool children. *Journal of Epidemiology and Community Health* **37**: 100–104.

Ward H, Norrie J, Sang A et al (1989) *Urban Safety Project: The Sheffield Scheme*. Contractors Report CR134. Crowthorne: Department of Transport Transport & Road Research Laboratory.

*Ward H, Cave J, Morrison A et al (1994) Pedestrian activity and accident risk. Basingstoke: AA Foundation for Road Safety Research.

West R, Sammons P & West A (1993) Effects of a traffic club on road safety knowledge and self-reported behaviour of young children and their parents. *Accident Analysis and Prevention* **25**: 609–618.

Williams AF & Wells JK (1981) Evaluation of the Rhode Island Child Restraint Law. *American Journal of Public Health* **71**: 742–743.

*Wilson MH, Baker SP, Tenet SP et al (1991) *Saving Children. A Guide to Injury Prevention*. Oxford: Oxford University Press.

5

Practitioners and policy makers

I. BARRY PLESS CM, MD, FRCP(C)

Professor
Departments of Pediatrics and Epidemiology & Biostatistics, McGill University, The Montreal Children's Hospital, 2300 Tupper Street, Room C-538, Montreal, Quebec H3H 1P3, Canada

ELIZABETH M. L. TOWNER* MA, BSc, PhD

Senior Lecturer in Community Child Health
Community Child Health, University of Newcastle upon Tyne, Donald Court House, 13 Walker Terrace, Gateshead NE8 1EB, UK

Unintentional injury in childhood is a major public health problem in all higher income countries and an increasing threat in many parts of the developing world. But it remains a relatively neglected aspect of health policy. This chapter explores what practitioners and policy makers can do to raise the profile of injury prevention on the local, national and international agenda. It examines the nature of childhood injuries and injury prevention that allows the field to be so neglected in health policies and considers why the public, professionals, and policy makers are unaware of the injury problem. The barriers that impede injury prevention programmes and research at the local level and that impede training in injury prevention for practitioners and policy makers are discussed. The development of the science and art of advocacy in injury prevention and the culture of safety are introduced. Examples of countries that have attempted to address the issues more actively are provided as lessons for practitioners and policy makers.

Key words: unintentional injury prevention; health policies; research; training; advocacy; culture of safety.

Unintentional injury in childhood is a major public health problem in all higher income countries and an increasing threat in many parts of the developing world (Manciaux and Romer, 1991). It is, therefore, surprising that injury prevention remains such a relatively neglected aspect of health policy. Perhaps as a reflection of this omission, it does not command funding for either programmes or research commensurate with the magnitude of the problem.

Why does this occur? What can practitioners and policy makers do to raise the profile of injury prevention on the local, national and international

* Author to whom all correspondance should be addressed.

Baillière's Clinical Paediatrics—
Vol. 5, No. 3, August 1997
ISBN 0–7020–2319–1
0963–6714/97/030393 + 15 $12.00/00

agenda? In this chapter we explore some of the reasons for the neglect of injury prevention, suggest potential solutions, provide examples of countries that have attempted to address the issue more actively, and, explore international developments in the field, and then consider what the lessons for practitioners or policy makers may be.

The American report *Injury Prevention: Meeting the Challenge*, which was published in 1989 noted that, 'practitioners often stumble over common obstacles, regardless of the community' (National Committee for Injury Prevention and Control, 1989). There are obstacles and challenges at every stage in the process, beginning with recognizing that injury is a problem, to finally institutionalizing solutions into a country's policy and infrastructure. To address these challenges, we first attempt to answer the following questions:

1. What is it about the nature of childhood injuries and injury prevention that allows the field to be so neglected in health policies?
2. Why are the public, professionals and policy makers unaware of the magnitude of the injury problem?
3. What barriers impede injury prevention programmes and research at the local level?
4. What barriers impede training in injury prevention for practitioners and policy makers?
5. How can the science and art of advocacy be promoted in injury prevention and the culture of safety developed?

WHAT IS IT ABOUT THE NATURE OF CHILDHOOD INJURIES AND INJURY PREVENTION THAT ALLOWS THE FIELD TO BE NEGLECTED IN HEALTH POLICIES?

Childhood unintentional injuries include a wide range of types of injury that occur in different environments. For example, the road environment includes pedestrians, passengers and bicyclists, while the home includes burns and scalds, poisonings, falls and asphyxiation. For each injury type a range of counter-measures is possible (Towner et al, 1996). One difficulty is that injuries occurring in different environments have been, historically, the responsibility of different agencies or government bodies, each of which may favour or advocate different approaches. Only when a public health approach is adopted are injuries viewed collectively as one disease and when this happens a more striking picture emerges. But prevention remains largely the remit of a range of agencies outside public health, e.g. transport, product safety, etc. A multi-disciplinary and multi-agency approach is thus needed and some form of lead agency must be designated to co-ordinate and oversee activities. Guyer and Gallagher, writing in 1985 in the USA, drew some interesting parallels between the development of the injury field and that of oncology; both had multi-disciplinary characteristics. Twenty years previously, individuals in different disciplines had approached the problem of cancer in an unco-ordinated manner; progress only occurred when the problem was redefined as one involving many disciplines (Guyer and Gallagher, 1985).

In the USA in particular, there has been much debate about the use of the term 'accident'. The concise Oxford English Dictionary defines an accident as 'An event that is without an apparent cause or an unexpected un-intentional act; chance; misfortune; unlucky event; especially one causing injury or damage'. The perception that injuries cannot be predicted or prevented may be, therefore, the most important barrier to progress in their prevention and control. When this view is held by policy makers it is especially likely to be counter-productive (Pless, 1991). Consequently, there is a need to demonstrate convincingly that injuries are not 'accidents'; that they are both predictable and preventable and, further, that they are subject to the same rules of inquiry as any other scientific discipline (Pless, 1991).

Another difficulty is that the field of injury prevention is likely to be perceived as 'worthy but dull'. Safety is likely to have a poor public image, especially in societies that promote and glorify risk-taking (National Committee for Injury Prevention and Control, 1989). Along similar lines, prevention of any kind is much less rewarding for practitioners than any form of cure because the successes of prevention are often impossible to measure. To add to these attitudinal problems, in many communities other values supersede the reduction of injury and it is thus difficult to motivate community members to learn about injuries and change their behaviour (National Committee for Injury Prevention and Control, 1989). Changing the climate of societal opinion takes time and requires a variety of comple-mentary approaches. For example, it took two decades to convince many Americans that drinking and driving is dangerous and not glamorous, yet many remain unconvinced or perceive that the problem is not one that affects them personally (National Committee for Injury Prevention and Control, 1989).

A more fundamental reason why injuries have not emerged as a major item on the health policy agenda of most countries is that other priorities dominate. Injury prevention is a relatively new field and does not have a natural lobby or advocacy group to promote it. Hence, there is no pressure on governments to acknowledge the importance of injury prevention. Moreover, in many countries, child health appears to be less important than health problems affecting adults, especially the elderly. Accordingly, child injury prevention is doubly disadvantaged when it competes with other health fields for priority or funding.

WHY ARE THE PUBLIC, PROFESSIONALS AND POLICY MAKERS UNAWARE OF THE MAGNITUDE OF THE INJURY PROBLEM?

It is quite likely that the answer to this question is similar to what was stated previously; as long as injuries are widely viewed as events that are not preventable or subject to proper scientific enquiry (e.g. 'accidents') the public as a whole, health professionals and policy makers will fail to respond to the injury problem in a manner that is consistent with its magnitude. It is one thing to say, 'yes, of course, many people die of accidents' but it is another to acknowledge that if this is so, the appropriate response should, logically, be no different than it is for any other public health problem. Thus, compounding the inappropriate response of the public is the failure of public health professionals in many countries to claim 'ownership' of the injury issue, or even to accept that it is part of their domain.

This view undoubtedly affects how the public perceives injury prevention. In addition, the media tend to focus on the more unusual, spectacular, or 'freak' accidents and ignore those that occur more frequently. They also fail to highlight the opportunities for prevention. For example, it is rare to see a report of a child car passenger who has been seriously injured in a crash but it is even rarer to find any mention of whether a suitable restraint was in use, or, if not, whether the parents have been appropriately penalized.

In countries where injury prevention receives more prominence, one reason this has been successfully achieved may be the provision of information about the cost of injuries relative to the cost of prevention. This strategy is often used to convince professionals and policy makers of the magnitude of the problem and its financial consequences compared to other causes of childhood ill health, many, if not most of which, cannot be prevented or cured.

WHAT BARRIERS IMPEDE INJURY PREVENTION PROGRAMMES AND RESEARCH AT A LOCAL LEVEL?

The first of these is the lack of good quality local data. This is discussed in greater length in Chapter 1. Vimpani (1989) has maintained that surveillance is one key to effective injury control. In countries where surveillance systems have been developed at a local or regional level, for example, Sweden, USA and Australia, generally more striking progress has been made in injury prevention. Surveillance data can be used in problem identification, to stimulate interest in the subject, to target specific injury types and localities, or to evaluate the impact of interventions. To illustrate the first of these, in South Australia, for example, examination of local surveillance data revealed that the risk of injury in children aged 2–12 years in bunk beds was almost five times that of children in conventional beds (Thompson, 1995). Further investigation of the data revealed that more than 10% of children fell from their bunk beds because of a structural failure. More than 10% fell when they were asleep, indicating inadequate rail design, and in 20% of the episodes the ladder was at fault. A survey of commercially available bunk beds confirmed the structural problems identified by the surveillance data. An Australian bunk bed standard was finally established after 4 years of lobbying and promotion and, eventually, safer bunk beds were manufactured.

Surveillance data can also be of value in educating the public, practitioners or policy makers about the size of the injury problem. Schelp (1988) describes the efforts made in a study in Falkoping to educate everyone, including local journalists about the problem of unintentional injury in the local area and motivating them to take a greater interest in injury prevention.

A second major barrier is the lack of information about effective interventions, although this is slowly being rectified. A World Health Organization report published in 1986 drew attention to the fact that despite the importance of unintentional injury there was a lack of evaluated studies on the effectiveness of injury prevention measures (WHO, 1986). In the decade since this report a number of reviews of effectiveness have been published and there has been considerable progress in the science and art of injury prevention (Bass et al, 1993; Pless, 1993; Towner et al, 1993, 1996; Klassen, 1995).

What the reviews reveal is that the published literature on interventions is not evenly spread over different injury types. In some areas there are numerous studies: the promotion of bicycle helmets or of child safety seats in cars being the most frequent. In other areas, such as the prevention of sports or leisure injuries, or drownings, few evaluation studies have been published (Towner et al, 1996).

Interventions that have been effective at reducing injury include a number of passive measures. These include child safety restraint legislation, child resistant closures to prevent poisoning, bicycle helmet legislation, area wide traffic calming measures, window guards to prevent falls and domestic product design. Examples of interventions that have been effective in changing behaviour include child restraint legislation, child restraint loan schemes, child restraint educational campaigns, bicycle helmet education and legislation, pedestrian education aimed at the child and/or the parent, provision of smoke detectors and parent education in hazard reduction (Towner et al, 1996).

Education, environmental modification and legislation all have a part to play and their effect in combination is important. Whether educational interventions are effective depend upon the context, the nature of the intervention, and whether it is suited to the target group. It also depends on the teaching methods employed (e.g. didactic or participative, the number of messages, the duration of the campaign, and whether significant groups, such as parents, are included). Some educational programmes have employed the use of rewards to foster significant behaviour changes. Educational campaigns in which a health professional e.g. a paediatrician, endorses the strategy, can be more effective. Examples include encouragement to use child safety restraints in cars, bicycle helmets, or smoke detectors (Bass et al, 1993).

Large scale environmental measures, such as area wide urban safety programmes, have been shown to reduce both pedestrian and bicycle injuries. Smaller scale product-based modifications, such as bicycle helmets, child safety restraints in cars, safe paraffin storage containers, can also be successful. Education promoting the use of such devices needs, however, to be reinforced by ensuring accessibility to the device, often by finding ways to reduce its cost. The technical adequacy of any such device or measure needs also to be sound. Legislation and regulation can offer a spectrum of protection, from single, one-off changes that offer passive protection to the child e.g. the design of washing machines to avoid chest scalds in young children, to measures that require repetitive action such as bicycle helmets or seatbelts in cars. The capacity to bring about environmental and legislative change is often based on modifying the climate of public opinion following educational campaigns (Towner et al, 1996). The issues of advocacy and a culture of safety are discussed later in this chapter.

As stated earlier, reviews of literature reveal many areas where there have been few evaluated interventions. These include studies to prevent sports and leisure injuries, and studies targeted at young adolescents, professionals and policy makers. The area of social deprivation also needs considerably more attention. Interventions relating to the alleviation of poverty or increasing social support need to be carefully evaluated. When new evaluation studies are planned it is important that they be well designed and include randomized control trials where appropriate. Good quality measures of non-fatal injury that include severity coding need to be developed and greater use could be made of 'intermediate' outcome measures such as risk data, for example, measuring the use of safety equipment by parents of pre-school children in different localities. To help replicate interventions that have produced positive results in other settings, process measures should always be reported in detail (Towner et al, 1996).

We know that a number of measures are effective and widespread application of what is known to be effective should be a high priority. When evidence of a measure or programme's efficacy is sufficiently compelling, there should follow immediate attempts to implement these measures as widely as possible (Pless, 1993). With increasing emphasis on effective health care and health promotion, policy makers need to be aware of what has been proved to work.

There is evidence that what is published in the research literature has little influence on the practice of child injury prevention. For example, a survey of practitioners in health and local authorities in England showed that education (including parental counselling) was the most commonly used type of prevention activity despite the scant support for this approach. In contrast, far fewer were involved with environmentally based interventions or those involving a safety device (Speller et al, 1995). A survey of nearly 1000 UK general practitioners also revealed that child injury prevention had failed to achieve widespread support in the primary care setting: 'It is practised to a varying extent by a minority of enthusiastic practitioners' ... and 'prevention advice tends to be offered opportunistically and sporadically rather than in a structured, age-specific manner' (Carter et al, 1995). A survey of head teachers of primary schools in Staffordshire, England, showed that although most felt that injury prevention was a suitable subject to be taught in schools, only a minority felt they had enough background information or training to teach the subject (Carter et al, 1994).

A major challenge exists to bridge the gap between research findings and actual practice. To do so, methods need to be found to disseminate research findings rapidly and ensure that they can be incorporated into practice guidelines, such as those of the American Academy of Pediatrics (AAP), or in the development of materials like the AAP's TIPP (The Injury Prevention Program) or the Australian ECIPP (Early Childhood Injury Prevention Program).

WHAT BARRIERS IMPEDE TRAINING IN INJURY PREVENTION FOR PRACTITIONERS AND POLICY MAKERS?

An unpublished survey by the International Paediatric Association reports that there is scarcely any training on injuries in medical faculties or in schools for allied health personnel, and what teaching there is almost always concentrates on the nature of the consequences of an accident rather than the epidemiological or preventive aspects (reported in Manciaux and Romer, 1991). In reviews of the effectiveness of injury prevention there are few examples of interventions that target the training of practitioners and even fewer of policy makers. The Falköping programme in Sweden was a notable exception; training and education of policy makers and health workers at the local level was a high priority. Resources were produced so that all district nurses had a home safety checklist to use on their visits to parents of young children (Schelp, 1988). A study from the USA on child care centres, directed at health professionals, aimed to change the culture and environment in the centres. For example, parents were encouraged to sign contracts agreeing to correctly restrain their children when they travelled in cars to and from the child care centres. Classroom activities for the children reinforced the seatbelt messages (Stuy et al, 1993)

In the USA the report *Injury Prevention: Meeting the Challenge* served as a resource for practitioners and would-be practitioners by providing statistics and practical advice to help them respond to the injury problem (National Committee for Injury Prevention and Control, 1989). In Australia, the Monash University Accident Research Centre aided the dissemination process by conducting short courses on injury research and prevention for professionals. The course held in 1991 was the first of its kind in Australia. For the second course, in 1994, a textbook was published, *Injury Research and Prevention: A Text*. It includes contributions from a range of disciplines and provides an overview for practitioners and academics in the injury field (Ozanne-Smith and Williams, 1995).

In summary, the barriers to training are, in part at least, the relative dearth of materials. But even with good material and texts of the kind described above, a fundamental barrier remains if injury prevention is not viewed by those responsible for training programmes as an element worthy of prominence. For all the reasons described earlier, this attitudinal barrier still exists, although in many countries it is being breached successfully.

HOW CAN THE SCIENCE AND ART OF ADVOCACY BE PROMOTED IN INJURY PREVENTION AND THE CULTURE OF SAFETY DEVELOPED?

Placing injury prevention higher on the agenda at the local, national, or international level requires advocacy to change public perceptions and move appropriate legislative action forward. Advocacy has a long tradition in both paediatrics and public health. Abraham Jacobi in his presidential address in 1889 at the founding of the American Pediatric Society proclaimed, 'the scientific attainments of the physician and his appreciation of the source of evil enabled him to strike at its roots by his advising aid and remedies' (reported in Christoffel and Runyan, 1995). Pediatricians have been behind many legislative initiatives to reduce injury (Grossman and Rivara, 1992). Notable examples are the introduction of child resistant containers in Britain, bicycle helmet legislation in Australia, and child safety restraint legislation in the USA. Case studies of how advocacy has been pursued are important; they serve as examples and inspiration for others who believe in the value of this strategy. But, as Robertson (1992) points out, 'Much of the research on laws focuses on the effects of enactment, enforcement or punishment; little research has been paid to how laws aimed at injury reduction are enacted'. The social and political processes that lead to enactment of or resistance to laws need to be carefully examined. Numerous observers have concluded that although solid data are important, as a rule, 'data alone are not enough to make policy makers act' (Christoffel and Runyan, 1995). Legislators are often more concerned about individual freedom, perceived constituent support and policy effectiveness (Lowenstein et al, 1993).

Nevertheless, data can be important: when child passenger safety bills were being considered by state legislatures the role of research information in influencing decisions was examined in a case study in Kansas and in a controlled experiment in Illinois (Fawcett et al, 1987). In the latter a package of information was sent to a randomly picked half of the senators in the experimental group but not sent to those in the control group. The study found that receiving the data positively affected the voting patterns of senators. Information on the frequency of the problem, the importance of child passenger safety, and the social acceptability of government legislation in this area, was also important and was used by the advocates (Fawcett et al, 1987).

Chapman and Lupton (1994) tried to analyse and describe the process of public health advocacy and to instruct potential practitioners in the skills involved. They describe a detailed case study from New South Wales in Australia of a protracted public battle involving advocacy for fencing to prevent childhood drownings in domestic swimming pools. In 1990 the Swimming Pool Fencing Act required existing private pools to have isolation fencing erected. Following 2 years of lobbying by pool owners opposed to this fencing, a new Act, the Swimming Pool Act of 1992, overturned this requirement. The ways in which the proponents and opponents of pool fencing framed their positions for the media are described by the authors.

The pro-fence group positioned themselves as protectors of the lives of small children. They stressed that to value votes, garden aesthetics, or avoiding financial outlay was the moral equivalent of infanticide. In contrast, the fence opponents stressed 'the backyard as a sanctuary from big brother', that individuals should fend for themselves, and that drownings resulted from negligent parenting. In the end, the latter argument succeeded in capturing public opinion and political will and the fence opponents won the political debate. On reflection, it appears the retrospective fencing demand in the first Act motivated considerable animosity and opposition by pool owners. A requirement for such fencing when a house is sold or a pool installed might have been more successful (Chapman and Lupton, 1994). Analysis of compelling examples such as this provide a strategic framework and foundation for the science as well as the art of advocacy.

The concept of 'a culture of safety' underlies much of what has been discussed in this chapter. Moller, in Australia, believes that such a culture influences what is known about injury and its causes, what is pursued as a priority, what is implemented, and what is considered to be effective (Moller, 1996). Within road safety, for example, engineering is the dominant profession and this has influenced the main solutions to road safety, namely, passive environmental strategies. In the past, drivers have been neglected in the problem solving exercise and only now are they, and other members of the local community being consulted by road safety engineers in local road design. Moller believes that more debate is needed 'about how the culture of safety can be shaped, the identification of the sources which shape it, and the development of strategies specifically targeted at developing a culture which is conducive to effective injury control' (Moller, 1996).

To foster advocacy and the safety culture examples of successes (and, perhaps, failures) need to be better publicized. At the same time, it is important to acknowledge that successful advocacy hinges on elements of personal style and not everyone can be expected to feel comfortable in this rôle. But for those who do, or think they might, there is only the examples of others to guide them. A few professional organizations have recently begun to offer seminars and workshops on advocacy; it is too soon to say how successful these have been.

As for the problem of cultural change, we now examine how three countries have, in their different ways, tackled this issue: Sweden, the USA and Australia. Here again, the purpose is to help others with similar goals learn by these examples.

SWEDEN

Sweden was the first to recognize the importance of injuries as a threat to child health and to tackle the problem in a co-ordinated manner. It has sustained this commitment to injury prevention for over 40 years. The Joint Committee for the Prevention of Accidents was formed in 1954, drawing membership from health and education services, safety organizations, professional groups and voluntary organizations (Berfenstam, 1979). It helped stimulate research, planning and regulations for a safer environment and provided information to parents and other key groups.

In 1957–59 Sweden had death rates from injuries in the 1–4 age group that were higher than the USA and those for the 5–14 age group were similar to those of the USA. However, by the late 1980s Sweden's childhood injury mortality rates were less than half those of the USA. In fact, it then had the lowest child injury death rates of any country in the world.

A variety of factors contributed to this resounding success: good surveillance data, a commitment to research, ensuring safer environments and products through regulation and legislation, and a broad-based safety education campaign using coalitions of existing groups (Bergman and Rivara, 1991). The charismatic and committed leadership of the joint committee was also significant. Three advocates of child safety, Ragnar Berfenstram, Theodore Ehrentreis and Ulla Bonde, met monthly for 25 years. The characteristics of Swedish society of homogeneity, prosperity and a sense of corporate responsibility meant that a culture of safety was nurtured. 'If a nation valued its children, their protection had to be a major societal goal. The safety of children had to be paramount when roads were built, products designed and buildings constructed'.

The source of funding for both practice and research is also significant. In Skaraborg county, for example, 50% of the health budget in the early 1990s was spent on health promotion and prevention. In other counties in Sweden the figure was between 10 and 30%. Because funds from biomedical research were limited, financial support for injury prevention was sought and obtained from insurance companies and car manufacturers (Bergman and Rivara, 1991).

USA

Most of the published papers in the English language on the epidemiology and prevention of childhood injuries come from the USA. One of the earliest attempts (starting in 1962) to systematically review injury prevention measures resulted in a list of ten counter-measures. These ranged from preventing the initial hazard to stabilizing, repairing and rehabilitating the damage (Haddon, 1980). This schema aided the process of thinking logically and non-categorically about injuries. Later, a landmark publication, *Injury in America* appeared (Committee on Trauma Research, Commission on Life Sciences and Medicine, 1985). It highlighted the problem, identified gaps in knowledge, and described the research needed to fill those gaps. Most importantly, it called on the US Congress to establish a centre for injury control within the federal government. The challenge was accepted and a pilot programme was established at the Centre of Disease Control (CDC) supported by $32 million in funding over a 3 year period. An early consequence was the establishment of five injury prevention research centres around the country.

After *Injury in America* was published, a conference of injury prevention professionals led to the writing of a book to serve as a resource for practitioners. *Injury Prevention: Meeting the Challenge* was thus prepared by the National Committee for Injury Prevention and Control in 1989. It was intended to help interested parties learn from and work with data, and to design, implement and evaluate interventions. By 1991 the CDC had convened seven injury control panels to develop position papers on setting a national agenda for injury control in the 1990s (Department of Health and Human Services, 1992).

In addition to funding for injury prevention and research from the federal government, the development of injury prevention coalitions at the local level was facilitated by a large grant from Johnson and Johnson, a pharmaceutical company, to establish the National 'Safe Kids' Campaign (Mickalide, 1995). This umbrella organization now, effectively, serves as principal spokesperson in childhood injury prevention issues in the USA. Although Safe Kids has many counterparts in other countries, the level of funding and the nature of its organization, makes it highly influential.

AUSTRALIA

In Australia, injuries have been recognized as important and preventable since the 1960s. The initial focus was on the road environment and later on occupational health. With the stimulus of the International Year of the Child in 1979, however, attention was drawn to childhood injury. The federal and state governments provided a grant of A$1 million to establish the Child Accident Prevention Foundation of Australia, now called Kidsafe (Albany and Kreisfeld, 1994).

The first composite picture of the nature and magnitude of injury as a health problem was drawn in 1986 when the Commonwealth Governments' report, *Looking Forward to Better Health* was published (Better Health Commission, 1986). Following from this a 4 year Better Health programme was established in 1988. In this programme, injury was identified as one of five priority areas and allocated 18% of the A$41 million committed to the programme as a whole. This stimulated activity at the national and state level. The National Injury Surveillance Unit (NISU) developed from a demonstration project, while, at the state level, important initiatives included the Victorian Injury Surveillance System, the Tasmanian Injury Surveillance and Research project, and an injury training course developed in South Australia (Albany and Kreisfeld, 1994)

Another important source of funding for injury prevention programmes in Australia are the health promotion foundations. These foundations receive funding from tobacco licensing fees and use these resources in the areas of health, sports and the arts. The Victoria Health Promotion Foundation, for example, has funded community-based programmes in the Shire of Bulla and Latrobe Valley as well as a public health training fellowship.

The scale and variety of sources of funding provided a great stimulus to progress in injury prevention in Australia and we can learn much from these successes. The Australian experience also provides lessons in the need to develop a solid infrastructure. Albany and Kreisfeld in their review of injury programmes and activities in Australia state that the national Better Health Programme 'fostered a significant number of short term projects which in the main were not subsequently absorbed into mainstream programmes and failed to reach maturity'. The failure to establish core injury prevention programmes at state and regional levels in the health sector meant that a body of expertise was not developed that would have lobbied 'to ensure the relocation of state public health resources from less strategic areas to that of injury prevention' (Albany and Kreisfeld, 1994).

INTERNATIONAL DEVELOPMENTS

It should come as no surprise that Sweden, the USA and Australia have been the most active promoters of injury prevention and control at the international level. These countries have hosted the first three meetings of the International Conference on Injury Prevention and Control and have been involved in the 'Safe Communities' network and conferences (Cohen, 1991). In addition, world conferences such as those in Ottawa, Canada in 1986 have reorientated health promotion, although of note is the fact that injury prevention as such was not among the main topics of discussion. A conference in Sundsvall, Sweden advocated the creation of supportive environments for health (Health and Welfare Canada, 1986; Sundsvall Conference on Special Environments, 1991).

In 1995, the first international society and journal devoted solely to the prevention of childhood injuries was launched. This was the International Society for Child and Adolescent Injury Prevention (ISCAIP) and its journal, *Injury Prevention*.

International links can be of great importance for committed groups in countries where there has been little interest in child injury prevention in the past. Although specific interventions are not necessarily generalizable from one country to another much can be learned from the successes and failures of other countries. Furthermore, recent efforts to establish a worldwide movement under the auspices of WHO are encouraging and should further help reluctant governments to address this issue more seriously.

WHAT ARE THE LESSONS FOR PRACTITIONERS AND POLICY MAKERS?

What has been learned about successes in child injury prevention are quite different for practitioners and policy makers. If a narrow definition of practitioners is applied, i.e. to refer only or mainly to health professionals, and more specifically, to physicians, the lessons are slim at best. There is some evidence that physician counselling is efficacious, i.e. that under ideal circumstances it can change behaviour of children or parents sufficiently to achieve substantially better prevention of injuries. But, effectiveness of physician education alone to achieve the same good results in the real world, seems highly doubtful. The main reason for this is logistics: those of time and resources, as well as other matters pertaining to how medical care is organized. Most physicians either do not have the time or are not willing to use what time they do have, for prevention activities, and injury prevention is no exception. In part this may be a reflection of reimbursement issues; when payment is based on a fee-for-item of service, prevention is likely to receive short shrift. But even in situations where capitation or straight salary is the rule, it is rare to find a physician inclined to spend much time on preventive counselling.

In contrast, nurses making home visits may be more effective at changing parent behaviours or the home surroundings. A meta-analysis (Roberts et al, 1996) suggests that of the relatively few such programmes that have been adequately evaluated, the result is usually quite positive. It is likely that success here hinges more on the opportunity to change the home environment than on parent education alone.

A final reason why physician couselling seems futile is that it is often necessary to inform parents not only about well-known hazards, such as poisons or the harm that may follow from inadequate or improper use of seat restraints or infant walkers, but also about new hazards, such as dangerous products. When monitoring or surveillance systems reveal such problems, it is foolish to believe that by notifying physicians the message will somehow find its way to all parents whose children are at risk. Even with computerized systems, that would permit doctors to identify all patients in specific, high-risk groups, e.g. by age, there is little reason to think that physicians would make a great effort to commit these resources to injury prevention. It would, in any case, be too little and, probably, too late.

Policy makers, on the other hand, once convinced of the value in doing so, have much more to offer, especially through enlightened legislation and regulations. A review of the major advances in injury prevention in childhood reveals that in each case a technological discovery or simply the creation or identification of a device or product, is the starting point for improved prevention. But the appropriate and widespread use of these devices, whether they be child resistant containers, child seat restraints, or bicycle helmets, is only likely to be achieved through the work of policy makers; specifically, through the passage of laws or the introduction of regulations. Legislating the use of child seat restraints resulted in an immediate increase in their rate of use in every country in which this has been studied. Similarly, regulations prohibiting the manufacture and sale of dangerous babywalkers resulted in their virtual elimination from the market in Canada, just as earlier regulations in Britain banning the use of drawstrings in children's clothing eliminated this cause of strangulations.

Regulations and laws require enforcement and the policy makers job is not done until the mechanisms are put in place for appropriate monitoring, detection and stringent punishment of violators. But the potential for prevention available to policy makers can never be underestimated. Thus, the issue for these key persons is to be convinced of the importance of acting in this arena. To persuade them, they must not only understand the magnitude of the problem, but also appreciate fully the extent to which these injuries are preventable.

REFERENCES

Albany P & Kreisfeld R (1994) *Injury Prevention and Control in Australia. A Review of Current Programs and Activities.* Canberra: Australian Government Publishing Service.

*Bass JL, Christoffel KK, Widome M et al (1993) Childhood injury prevention counseling in primary care settings: a critical review of the literature. *Pediatrics* **92:** 544–550.

Berfenstam R (1979) Prevention of childhood accidents in Sweden with special attention to the work of the Joint Committee for Prevention of Accidents. *Acta Paediatrica Scandinavica* **275 (Supplement):** S88–S95.

Bergman A & Rivara F (1991) Sweden's experience in reducing childhood injuries. *Pediatrics* **88:** 69–74.

Better Health Commission (1986) *Looking Forward to Better Health.* Canberra: Australian Government Publishing Service.

Carter Y, Bannon M & Jones P (1994) The role of the teacher in child accident prevention. *Journal of Public Health Medicine* **16:** 23–28.

Carter Y, Morgan P & Lancashire RJ (1995) General practitioners' attitudes to child injury prevention in the UK: a national postal questionnaire. *Injury Prevention*, **1:** 164–167.

*Chapman S & Lupton D (1994) *The Fight for Public Health. Principles and Practice of Media Advocacy.* London: BMJ Publishing Group.

*Christoffel K & Runyan C (1995) *Adolescent Injuries: Epidemiology and Prevention. State of the Art Reviews.* Vol. 6. Philadelphia: Hanley and Belfus.

Cohen D (1991) Manifesto for safe communities. *Medical Journal of Australia* **154:** 302–303 (Commentary).

*Committee on Trauma Research, Commission on Life Sciences and Medicine, National Research Council Institute of Medicine (1985) *Injury in America: A Continuing Public Health Problem.* Washington, DC: National Academic Press.

Department of Health and Human Services (1992) *Setting the National Agenda for Injury Control in the 1990's.* Position Papers from the Third National Injury Control Conference, Denver, Colorado, April 1991.

Fawcett S, Seekins T & Jason L (1987) Policy research and child passenger safety legislation: a case study and experimental evaluation. *Journal of Social Issues* **43:** 133–148.

Grossman D & Rivara F (1992) Injury control in childhood. *Pediatric Clinics of North America* **39:** 5–15

Guyer B & Gallagher S (1985) An approach to the epidemiology of childhood injuries. *Pediatric Clinics of North America*, **32:** 5–15.

*Haddon W (1980) Advances in the epidemiology of injuries as a basis for public policy. *Public Health Reports* **95:** 411–421.

Health and Welfare Canada (1986) *Ottawa Charter for Health Promotion, and Conference on Health Promotion: The Move Towards a New Public Health.* Ottawa, Canada, November 1986.

Klassen T (1995) *The effectiveness of injury control interventions.*, MSc thesis, McMaster University, Hamilton, Ontario, Canada.

Lowenstein S, Koziol-McLain J, Scatterfield G et al (1993) Facts versus values: why legislators vote against injury control laws. *Journal of Trauma*, **35:** 786.

*Manciaux M & Romer CJ (eds) (1991) *Accidents in Childhood and Adolscence. The Role of Research.* Geneva: World Health Organisation.

Mickalide A (1995) The National 'Safe Kids' Campaign (USA). *Injury Prevention* **1:** 119–121.

Moller J (1996) The culture of safety: a foundation for envrionmental and behavioural change. Paper presented at the Third International Conference on Injury Prevention and Control, Melbourne, Australia, February 1996.

*National Committee for Injury Prevention and Control (1989) *Injury Prevention: Meeting the Challenge.* New York: Oxford University Press.

Ozanne-Smith J & Williams F (eds) (1995) *Injury Research and Prevention: A Text*. Victoria, Australia: Monash University Accident Research Centre (MUARC).

*Pless IB (1991) Accident Prevention. *British Medical Journal*, **303**: 462–464.

Pless IB (1993) *The Scientific Basis of Childhood Injury Prevention. A Review of the Medical Literature*. London: Child Accident Prevention Trust.

*Roberts I, Kramer M & Suissa S (1996) Does home visiting prevent childhood injury? A systematic review of randomised controlled trials. *British Medical Journal* **312**: 29–33.

Robertson LS (1992) *Injury Epidemiology*. New York: Oxford University Press.

Schelp L (1988) The role of organizations in community participation—prevention of accidental injuries in a rural Swedish municipality. *Social Science and Medicine* **26**: 1087–1093.

Speller V, Mulligan J, Law C & Foot B (1995) *Preventing Injury in Children and Young People. A Review of the Literature and Current Practice Report*. Winchester: Wessex Institute of Public Health Medicine.

Stuy M, Green M & Doll J (1993) Child care centres: a community resource for injury prevention. *Developmental and Behavioral Pediatrics*, **14**: 224–229.

Sundsvall Conference On Special Environments (1991) Playing For Time: Creating Supportive Environments for Health. Paper presented at the Third International Conference on Health Promotion, Sundsvall, Sweden, June 1991.

Thompson P (1995) Bunk beds: classic example of a prevention strategy. In Ozanne-Smith J & Williams F (eds) *Injury Research and Prevention: A Text*, pp 197–201. Victoria, Australia: Monash University Accident Research Centre (MUARC).

Towner E, Jarvis S, & Dowswell T (1993) *Reducing Childhood Accidents. The Effectiveness of Health Promotion Interventions: A Literature Review*. London: Health Education Authority.

*Towner E, Dowswell T, Simpson G & Jarvis S (1996) *Health Promotion in Childhood and Young Adolescence for the Prevention of Unintentional Injuries*, vol. 1. London: Health Education Authority.

Vimpani G (1989) Injury Surveillance: a key to effective control of childhood injuries. *Australian Paediatric Journal* **25**: 890–893

WHO (World Health Organisation) (1986) *Accidents in Children and Young People*, vol. 39. Geneva: WHO.

6

Immediate management of the injured child

KEITH M. PORTER FRCS, DipIMC, RCS(Ed)

Consultant Trauma and Orthopaedic Surgeon
Selly Oak Hospital, Raddlebarn Road, Birmingham B29 6JD, UK

SEAN WALSH MRCPI, MSc, DCH

Consultant in Accident and Emergency Medicine
Leeds General Infirmary, Great George Street, Leeds LS1 3EX, UK

The treament of seriously injured children should be optimum from the earliest stages in order to reduce further morbidity and mortality. This involves a structured approach that applies to both pre-hospital care and hospital care.

Medical treatment is focused on early identification and treatment of life threatening injuries. This involves a rapid assessment, based on the injured child's ABC (airway, breathing and circulation) with the ability to intervene and correct problems as they are identified.

This approach is further supplemented by a full head to toe examination of the child, to ensure all injuries are identified. Finally, a definitive medical care plan can be instituted for the individual child.

Key words: resuscitation; trauma; pre-hospital.

Trauma is the commonest cause of death between the ages of 1 and 15, with head injury being the commonest single cause of death. Road accident victims constitute the main group followed by burns and falls in order of frequency. Deaths from trauma follow a trimodal distribution. The immediate deaths are those that are instantaneous or occur within minutes of the accident and include patients suffering airway obstruction and catastrophic external haemorrhage.

The second group includes patients with unrecognized or untreated hypoxia and hypovolaemia particularly from chest injuries and abdominal trauma and also includes unrecognized intracranial complications. These occur within hours of the accident and with appropriate treatment and intervention some deaths can be avoided. The final group includes deaths occurring weeks after the accident and includes patients dying of infection and multiple organ system failure. Audit has shown in some of these late deaths that there was a delay in resuscitation and in some cases diagnosis and treatment.

Baillière's Clinical Paediatrics —
Vol. 5, No. 3, August 1997
ISBN 0–7020–2319–1
0963–6714/97/030409 + 11 $12.00/00

409

Current management of paediatric trauma is based on principles laid out in the *Advanced Trauma Life Support* (ATLS) *Course Core Course Manual* (American College of Surgeons, 1988) and in *Advanced Paediatric Life Support* (APLS) (Advanced Life Support Group, 1993) courses. These can be applied with appropriate modification in both pre-hospital and hospital settings. An important element common to both is the need for a 'team' approach from medical personnel dealing with injured children.

PREPARATION AND APPROACH TO THE SCENE

A doctor may come across an accident by chance or be part of a British Association of Immediate Care (BASICS) Scheme and be tasked by the local ambulance control to attend an injured child. Infrequently a hospital flying squad may be mobilized for their specific expertise.

The BASICS doctor, as a matter of routine, should ensure that his vehicle is in working order, appropriately maintained and his equipment is complete and his drugs are in date. The doctor should drive safely and appropriately to the scene using a green rotating beacon as a visible warning device and, where local arrangements exist, an audible warning system. On arrival at the scene he should put on his personal protective clothing which should be a yellow-green fluorescent jacket, positively identifying him as a 'doctor'. Gloves should always be worn. On arrival the doctor should log in with ambulance control as a matter of routine.

Safety is the first priority and includes safety of the scene, safety of the carer and safety of the patient. Scene safety includes protection from on-coming traffic, recognition of a fire risk, risk of electric shock, dangerous chemicals or gases and dangers from unstable vehicles or unstable buildings etc.

As a general principle the doctor should not rush head long into the incident and should inspect the scene carefully and methodically so as to get an overall picture. Specifically the doctor should make contact as soon as possible with the ambulance crews in attendance and liaise with the senior ambulance, police and fire officers present.

The doctor should ascertain exactly what has happened, the nature of the incident, how many casualties there are, the type of injuries involved, how severely injured are the patients and whether the patients are trapped. He should have information about any specific hazards as well as any potential access problems. The doctor, in conjunction with the ambulance service, should ensure when necessary that the other services have been alerted, and determine whether specific medical or ambulance service back-up in the form of more extended skills trained paramedics or accredited BASICS doctors are needed. Consideration should be given to the mode of transportation, which may be by land ambulance or by helicopter and to the chosen receiving hospital. It is important to get the right patient to the right hospital at the right time.

Inspection of the wreckage will allow an experienced immediate care doctor to 'read the wreckage' and predict patterns of injury based on both exterior and interior damage including intrusion deformity. It should be noted that in the case of a pedestrian struck by a car a small child will sustain injuries to his pelvis or chest and not the usual bumper injuries sustained by adults simply because of the child's short stature.

The attending doctor should not interfere unnecessarily with any debris or wreckage at the scene as this may require inspection by the police for forensic purposes at a later time.

Consideration should be given to searching for ejected or unaccounted casualties whose presence may not be obvious to begin with. A baby's car seat may alert the rescuer to the possibility of a small child either ejected from the vehicle or trapped deep within the wreckage.

APPROACH TO THE PATIENT

Initial priority should be to treat those patients who will die unless treated immediately and this includes opening the obstructed airway and the control of major external haemorrhage. A systematic and structured approach is necessary in order to identify and treat problems in order of priority. The Advanced Trauma Life Support (ATLS) philosophy has introduced a structured approach to patient care, based on the following four steps:

- Primary survey.
- Resuscitation.
- Secondary survey.
- Definitive care.

Pre-hospital care may involve a primary survey and resuscitation only. It may not be appropriate or indeed there may not be time to undertake even a limited secondary survey, in which case a detailed secondary survey and definitive care plan is the remit of the accident and emergency department.

Primary survey

Life threatening problems are recognized during the primary survey (based on an ABCDE approach) and this system should be applied to all patients regardless of the causation and mechanism of injury.

A, Airway and cervical spine control.
B, Breathing.
C, Circulation and control of external haemorrhage.
D, Disability.
E, Exposure and environment.

Any problem identified during the primary survey is immediately rectified before moving on to the next assessment point. For instance, an airway problem is rectified before reviewing breathing and should a breathing problem be identified such as an open pneumothorax, this is rectified before undertaking a circulatory assessment.

Environment is added to exposure because of the significant risk of hypothermia in the injured child, particularly the smaller child, especially if the child is exposed to the elements for any period of time during assessment and treatment or in an entrapment situation.

A, Airway and cervical spine

Initial approach to the patient should include placing a hand on the forehead and then gently shaking the child's arm and asking the child 'Are you all right?' If the child is able to respond and talk, this implies a patent airway.

Cervical spine injury should be assumed to be present in all victims of trauma who are rendered unconscious or who have been unconscious and in all who have evidence of an injury above the clavicles. For this reason the airway opening manoeuvre should be the jaw thrust procedure rather than a chin lift and head tilt. Opening the airway is of greater priority than cervical spine control. If the airway can only be opened by a small amount of head tilt then this should be undertaken. Without an open airway the child will rapidly die from hypoxia quickly. It is noted that the airway is opened in the infant in the neutral position and in the child in the sniffing position.

Any obvious foreign bodies should be removed, though a finger sweep is contra-indicated for fear of pushing any debris or foreign object further down the airway. If airway obstruction persists then consider an oropharangeal or a naso-pharangeal airway. The latter, whilst potentially contra-indicated in fractures of the base of the skull, may be the only means of opening an airway particularly in the child having sustained a head injury who clenches his teeth together. If airway obstructions persist then consider intubation and if this in turn is unsuccessful then consider a cricothyroidotomy. Ideally in line cervical stabilization should be maintained by a second person at all times.

B, Breathing

Breathing should be assessed once the airway has been opened and the cervical spine controlled.

The chest should be exposed irrespective of the environment. The chest should be inspected for chest movement particularly symmetry of chest movements, evidence of any open pneumothorax or flail chest demonstrated by paradoxical chest movements. The rescuer should quickly feel the back of the chest, without moving the patient, with his gloved hand and look for any blood indicative of posterior wounds. Respiratory rate should be assessed and the chest auscultated and percussed to determine dullness, increased resonance and air entry. In addition the central position of the trachea should be confirmed and the neck veins assessed for distension.

A tension pneumothorax occurs when air accumulates under pressure in the pleural space and pushes the mediastinum across the chest restricting venous return to the heart and cardiac output is reduced. The child will be hypoxic and may be shocked. There is decreased air entry and hyper-resonance on the side of the tension pneumothorax. There may be visible distended neck veins and as a late physical sign the trachea will deviate away from the side of the tension pneumothorax. The tension pneumothorax is relieved by a needle thoracocentesis and the child given high flow oxygen therapy through a reservoir bag and non-rebreathing system. Ultimately, the child will require a chest drain placement on the affected side. The use of a bag valve mask system or indeed intubation and positive pressure ventilation may convert a previously unrecognized simple pneumothorax into a tension pneumothorax. Neck vein distention will not occur in the shocked hypovolaemic patient.

An open pneumothorax is a penetrating wound to the chest wall usually from outside in. Air may be noted blowing or sucking through the wound. Treatment involves sealing the wound and securing a dressing on three sides allowing air to escape on the non-sealed side should tension build up within. This manoeuvre will now stop air from sucking into the chest and will allow some degree of ventilation of the underlying lung. Patients should receive high flow oxygen as in all chest injuries. Within hospital a chest drain can be sited to treat the underlying pneumothorax.

Flail chest—a child's chest, particularly the young child, is extremely compliant and therefore rib fractures and flail segments are a rare occurrence except in severe kinetic energy transfer usually associated with falls and road traffic accidents. The child will be hypoxic (due to pulmonary contusions) and there may be evidence of paradoxical respiration, palpable rib crepitus, although initially the child may successfully splint his chest. An obvious flail segment should be stabilized manually with the flat of the hand, which reduces pain and importantly obliterates the paradoxical movement and will allow a negative intrathoracic pressure to occur prior to inspiration and, therefore, ventilation of the underlying lung. The chest may also be stabilized by strapping a 500 cc bag of saline to the chest wall or by appropriate positioning of the child with their injured side lying on a firm object.

Massive haemothorax occurs due to damage to the lung parenchyma and occasionally great vessels. The child will be in shock and on the side of the haemothorax there will be decreased chest movements, dullness to percussion and absent or decreased breath sounds. Treatment involves high flow oxygen therapy and transfer to hospital urgently. Depending on the journey time to hospital intravenous access may be gained en route to hospital. On arrival at hospital the child will need a chest drain to evacuate the blood and improve ventilation.

Cardiac tamponade is most commonly seen following penetrating trauma as a consequence of a collection of blood in the pericardial sac. Cardiac output is compromised. The child will be in shock and the neck veins may be distended, although this may not be obvious if hypovolaemia is also present. Heart sounds are muffled, although at a road traffic accident, for instance, it may be difficult to hear anything other than the ambient noise and it may not be until the child is moved into the ambulance that extraneous noise is sufficiently decreased to allow adequate cardiac auscultation. Treatment includes oxygen therapy, intravenous access depending on the time to hospital and those trained in pre-hospital care and paediatric resuscitation should consider undertaking emergency needle pericardiocentesis. A small volume of blood removed from the pericardial sac can dramatically improve the clinical position. Within the hospital setting, these children will require consultation with Paediatric Cardio-thoracic Surgeons.

Diaphragmatic rupture is usually associated with blunt trauma to the abdomen and almost invariably occurs on the left side. Physical signs usually become apparent some time after the accident.

The optimal position to allow adequate ventilation and perfusion of an injured lung is with the injured lung uppermost and the patient lying on their non-injured side. Whether to adopt this position or not will be governed by other priorities and circumstances.

The normal resting respiratory rate varies in children as does the pulse and blood pressure and these are summarized in Table 1. Most children requiring breathing support in the pre-hospital scene can be adequately managed using a bag valve mask and reservoir bag system.

Table 1. Normal vital signs in childhood.

Age	Respiratory rate	Systolic blood pressure	Pulse
<1	30–40	70–90	110–160
2–5	25–30	80–100	95–140
5–12	20–25	90–110	80–120
>12	15–20	100–120	60–100

C, Circulation and control of external haemorrhage

Circulation is initially assessed by checking peripheral and central pulses. A radial pulse is indicative of essential organ perfusion. Any obvious external bleeding should be controlled by the simplest method that will stem the haemorrhage. This includes in order of progression: direct pressure, elevation, pressure points—and if there is still uncontrolled life threatening haemorrhage from a limb injury, the application of a tourniquet.

Should it be necessary to use a tourniquet the time of application should be noted, and its presence and time of application made clear to the receiving hospital on the patient's arrival.

Immobilization of limb fractures, whether opened or closed, will reduce blood loss. Haemorrhage from large flap scalp lacerations may be controlled by using a hair tie or turning the flap inside out and then apply-ing direct pressure. Except in infants where blood loss from the scalp injury can be excessive, hypotension in trauma is never associated with an isolated head or scalp injury.

Besides determining the presence or absence of peripheral pulses and the heart rate the circulatory status can be further assessed by pulse volume, capillary refill time, skin temperature, respiratory rate and the mental status. Increased respiratory rate in the absence of a chest injury is an early indicator of hypovolaemia. Mental agitation and changes in the level of consciousness can be compromised by primary brain injury and also associated hypoxia due to chest injuries.

Capillary refill time is tested by pressing for 5 seconds over the nail bed and the normal colour should return within 2 seconds. Capillary refill time may be prolonged in the cold and comparison should then be made to the capillary refill time of the rescuer.

Assessment of observed clinical parameters provides an estimate of percentage of blood loss (Table 2).

Table 2. Physiological responses to blood loss in childhood.

	Blood loss (%)		
	Up to 25%	25–40%	>40%
Heart rate	Increased+	Increased++	Increased+++ or bradycardia
Systolic blood pressure	Normal	Normal or falling	Falling+++
Pulse volume	Normal or decreased	Decreased+	Decreased++
Capillary refill	Normal/increased	Increased+	Increased++
Skin temperature	Cool, pale	Cold	Cold
Respiratory rate	Increased+	Increased++	Sighing respiration
Mental state	Normal or agitated	Drowsy, uncooperative	Unconscious

In infants the brachial or femoral artery should be palpated in view of the difficulty in feeling the carotid pulse because of their short fat necks. Should the pulse rate be less than 60 beats/minute in infants and small children and less then 40 beats/minute in larger children then cardiac compressions are required.

The shocked and hypotensive child in the pre-hospital environment cannot normally be stabilized and has a surgical lesion, such as a major intrathoracic or intra-abdominal bleed. Out of hospital interventions should be limited to opening the airway, ensuring adequate breathing and, if necessary, ventilation, arresting any obvious external bleeding and rapid transfer to hospital. Depending on the journey time it may be appropriate to obtain vascular access en route to hospital. There should be no delay at the scene in attempting to gain vascular access. Attempting to place a drip in the cold, damp and dark environment, perhaps in a vehicle with a trapped child is difficult and experienced pre-hospital care practitioners will verify that the simplest means of vascular access is an interosseous needle. This should be the vascular access route of choice under these circumstances.

Within the accident and emergency department, children with hypo-tension following trauma need intravenous access and fluid replacement. Fluid replacement should initially be 20 ml of crystalloid/kilogram body weight, depending on response, followed by 20 ml of colloid/kilogram. If there is an inadequate response to this, then blood transfusion at 10–20 ml/kilogram should be commenced and an urgent surgical opinion/ intervention obtained (Yurt, 1992).

If there is no obvious source for the blood loss externally, then the attending doctor needs to keep a high level of suspicion for an intra-abdominal or intrathoracic source. The use of ultrasound and computed tomography (CT) scan imaging may assist in diagnosis (Morton and Phillips, 1996).

D, Disability

Assessment of neurological status during the primary survey involves a brief neurological examination to determine pupillary size and reaction and an assessment on the AVPU score.

A = Alert
V = Responds to voice
P = Responds to pain
U = Unconsciousness

The use of more detailed methods of ascertaining level of consciousness, such as the Glasgow Coma Scale can be performed later as part of the Secondary Survey.

E, Exposure and environment

Exposure should be adequate to ensure recognition of life threatening injuries and this, in particular, includes adequate chest exposure. However, at the same time a child should be protected from the environment, particularly cold, damp and wet and also protected from hypothermia. The injured child should not be moved from the position where they are found unless there is imminent danger, and should be assessed and treated where found pending the arrival of the emergency services.

When children are transported to hospital, it is important to realize that they still are prone to hypothermia if they have prolonged times of exposure.

RESUSCITATION

Resuscitative measures are undertaken as soon as a problem is identified in the primary survey and, therefore, in this respect resuscitation merges into the primary survey. Resuscitation involves life saving interventions including opening and securing an airway, administration of high flow oxygen through a non-rebreathing bag with a reservoir mask, cervical spine control and stabilization, ensuring adequate breathing and where necessary ventilation, the recognition and treatment of life threatening emergencies including open pneumothoraces, tension pneumothoraces, flail chests and cardiac tamponade and also the arrest of obvious external bleeding.

Within the accident and emergency department, these resuscitation measures are reassessed and continued as appropriate. In addition, vascular access in the form of two periphal lines are initiated. Blood samples for full blood count, electrolytes, glucose and cross-matching are taken and sent.

Thereafter, the child should have X-rays taken of the lateral cervical spine, chest, pelvis and other areas (e.g. skull, limbs) as appropriate.

Finally, the child should have an orogastric tube and urinary catheter sited.

SECONDARY SURVEY

Following the primary survey and resuscitation in a stable patient a secondary survey may be undertaken. In time-critical injuries this should be undertaken in the accident and emergency department. The secondary survey is essentially a head to toe examination in an anatomical and methodical way. The secondary survey should involve recognizing non-life threatening injuries and potential complications.

Head injury

Any scalp bleeding not previously controlled or recognized should receive an appropriate dressing. The ears and the nose should be inspected for a CSF leak. The patient should be re-assessed on the AVPU scale and pupillary reaction again recorded. The child can also be scored on the Glasgow Coma Scale or the Children's Coma Scale. The object of management involves the prevention of secondary brain damage, which is invariably associated with hypoxia and hypovolaemia. Cerebral perfusion pressure is equal to the mean systemic blood pressure minus the mean intracranial pressure.

Blood pressure may be maintained by controlling external bleeding and also elevating the legs and, where time permits, judicious fluid replacement. Intracranial pressure is influenced by the maintenance of adequate oxygenation and the prevention of hypercapnia. If a child requires assisted ventilation then hyperventilation will help reduce cerebral oedema. Other interventions such as intubation and infusion of mannitol are normally reserved for hospital management.

The uncooperative child who may be confused and perhaps combative following a head injury cannot be appropriately immobilized using a collar and spinal board and should be supported as best as possible and, if possible, a cervical collar in isolation fitted, though again this may prove impossible. A combative patient is likely to do more harm to themselves than to co-operate with carers advice. Beware of the hypoxic and hypovolaemic patient who can present with exactly this scenario.

Facial trauma

The facial skeleton should be examined for any obvious deformity or lacerations and the inside of the mouth examined for any previously unrecognized bleeding and any obvious loose teeth.

Neck examination

The cervical collar if previously applied should not be disturbed. Detailed physical examination of the neck should take place after appropriate radiology in the accident and emergency department.

Chest examination

The chest should be further examined for evidence of external injury in the form of bruising crepitus and surgical emphysema implying an internal air leak. In addition the trachea should again be checked and the chest palpalted and auscultated to determine evidence of haemothorax and pneumothorax.

Abdominal examination

The abdomen should be inspected for evidence of bruising and wounds and palpated for tenderness, rigidity and guarding. If present they are the hall-marks of internal injury. A specific diagnosis is not necessary. Recognizing a potential surgical abdomen and the prompt need for transfer to hospital is essential.

Pelvic examination

The pelvic girdle should be examined for any bruising and any pain or crepitus on pelvic springing. Inspection of the urinary meatus and perineum should be undertaken in hospital.

Spinal injuries

Inspection of the spine involves a formal log roll and this should be undertaken during the secondary survey in the accident and emergency department.

Extremity trauma

Limbs are inspected and palpated looking for evidence of bruising, swelling, deformity and crepitus. Obvious fractured limbs are not moved. It is important to assess the peripheral sensation and circulation. Limb splintage may reduce pain and will also reduce fracture blood loss.

In the absence of significant external haemorrhage associated with open fractures evaluation is carried out during the secondary survey and in time-critical injury may well be delayed until arrival at hospital. Multiple fractures can produce hypovolaemia, and blood loss is minimized even in closed fractures by appropriate splintage. Closed femoral fractures can bleed up to 20% of circulatory volume and an open fracture up to 40% loss which is a life threatening scenario.

Distal circulation and sensation should be assessed where possible. Compartmental syndrome related to increased swelling within anatomical compartments does not usually develop until several hours after injury and is not normally a recognized pre-hospital problem. Analgesia including Entonox (unless contra-indicated) or intravenous opiates are appropriate analgesics. Femoral nerve blocks are very effective in pain relief in femoral fracture and can be undertaken in a pre-hospital setting.

DEFINITIVE CARE

Once the child has been adequately resuscitated and stabilized, a management plan that incorporates further investigations and treatment can be formalized. The exact nature of this will focus on prioritizing the injuries in terms of 'threat to life' and will also depend on the facilities and medical expertise available in the individual hospital. (Moront et al, 1994).

TRANSPORT TO HOSPITAL

Most patients will be formally 'packaged', which will include spinal boarding with head huggers and appropriate monitoring including ECG monitoring and pulse oximetry. During transportation to hospital any deterioration in the patient's clinical state warrants a return to the primary survey and an ABC examination.

Pulse oximetry, whilst a valuable monitoring adjunct, can record a normal PO_2 with supplementary oxygen yet the patient may be hypoventilating and becoming hypercarbic. Furthermore pulse oximetry is unreliable in the cold, shut-down patient, patients wearing nail varnish, the anaemic patient and in patients with carbon monoxide poisoning.

The receiving hospital should be kept informed of the condition of the child, the estimated time of arrival and the response required from the hospital, i.e., trauma team, anaesthetist, surgeon, etc.

If the child is to be transferred between hospitals for ongoing care, it is important that suitably trained staff accompany the child. If the child has been intubated and ventilated an anaesthetist must be part of the Transfer team. In addition the correct equipment along with suitable drugs and fluid therapies must be readily available during transfer.

REFERENCES

Advanced Life Support Group (1993) *Advanced Paediatric Life Support—The Practical Approach.* London: BMJ.

American College of Surgeons (1988) *Advanced Trauma Life Support Course Core Course Manual.* Chicago, IL: American College of Surgeons.

Moront M, Williams J, Eichelberger M et al (1994) The injured child—an approach to care. *Paediatric Clinics of North America* **41:** 1201–1226.

Morton R & Phillips B (eds) (1996) *Accidents and Emergencies in Children.* Oxford: Oxford University Press.

Yurt R (1992) Triage, initial assessment, and early treatment of the paediatric trauma patient. *Paediatric Clinics of North America* **39:** 1083–1091.

7

Do we need trauma centres?

JANETTE K. TURNER BSc, RN

Research Fellow

JONATHON P. NICHOLL BA, MSc, CStat, HonMFPHM

Director

Medical Care Research Unit, University of Sheffield, Regent Court, 30 Regent Street, Sheffield S1 4DA, UK

BARBARA M. PHILLIPS FRCP, FFAEM

Consultant in Paediatric Emergency Medicine
Accident and Emergency Department, Alder Hey Children's Hospital, Eaton Road, Liverpool L12 2AP, UK

The aim of a trauma service should be to provide care which maximizes the chances of survival and minimizes consequent morbidity. This is best achieved by designing a system of care that is responsive to the needs of any given trauma population. The characteristics of paediatric trauma populations can be described in terms of injury patterns and mechanisms, volumes and the response to injury. In the USA the predominant trauma care model is that of regionalized trauma systems containing specialist trauma centres. In the UK paediatric trauma accounts for a much smaller proportion of hospital workload and hence an alternative system of care may be more appropriate. In this chapter the research evidence of the impact of different trauma system designs on patient outcome is reviewed and some suggestions are given on how pre-hospital and acute hospital services for paediatric trauma could be organized in the UK.

Key words: injury; health service needs and demand; trauma centres; children; mortality; injury epidemiology; outcome.

Injury has always been, and continues to be a major cause of mortality in children. In the USA in 1995 39% of deaths in children were the result of trauma and accounted for more childhood deaths than all other causes combined (Rosenberg et al, 1996). In the UK just under 10% of all deaths in children are due to trauma, 27% in the 1–14 years group (Office for National Statistics, 1996).

Child mortality due to accidents has fallen dramatically during this century. Nevertheless injury continues to be a significant cause of

Baillière's Clinical Paediatrics—
Vol. 5, No. 3, August 1997
ISBN 0–7020–2319–1
0963–6714/97/030421 + 13 $12.00/00

morbidity and mortality with consequent demands on health care resources and is seen as a priority area for further reduction (DoH, 1991).

This chapter examines how the organization and delivery of trauma services can contribute to improving outcome following injury in the paediatric population. Clearly there is no one 'best way' of achieving this. Different populations have different needs and the services most likely to have an impact on outcome are those that have been designed to respond to the characteristics of the population they serve. Much of the information we draw upon is from studies in the USA where trauma system development has been progressing since the 1970s. However these systems are not necessarily directly transferable to other settings. So, although consideration will be given to USA trauma system designs, conclusions about the need for trauma centres have been made in the light of the nature of paediatric trauma in the UK.

THE EPIDEMIOLOGY OF PAEDIATRIC TRAUMA

Injury patterns

Children sustain the same types of injury as adults but there are differences in the relationship between injury type and cause of death (Table 1).

Table 1. UK causes of death due to injury.

Cause of deaths (%)		Child (0–14 yrs)	Adult
% of all UK deaths due to trauma	0–14 years	8.2	
	1–14 years	27	2.2
Head		52.6	25.7
Internal Injury of abdomen/chest/pelvis		18	19.5
Fractures (other than skull)		2.5	25.9
Burns		4.1	2.6
Drowning		7.8	4.8
Asphyxiation/strangulation		10.4	13.8
Others		4.6	7.7

Source: Office of National Statistics (1996).

Head injury predominates in all trauma populations and, in general, is the leading cause of trauma death although there are some small regional variations. In some American states the effects of fire, usually associated with urban poverty, account for the largest proportion of trauma deaths in children (Hall et al, 1993).

Skeletal injuries are the second most common type of injury but are much more likely to be a cause of death in adults where complications associated with fractured femur account for a large number of deaths in the elderly. Internal injuries of the chest, abdomen and pelvis account for the same proportion of trauma deaths in adults and children.

A more detailed picture of injury types for all paediatric major trauma (Injury Severity Score (ISS) > 15) in a UK population is given in Table 2. The data is taken from a large study that evaluated the cost-effectiveness of an experimental regionalized trauma system (Nicholl et al, 1995). Patient outcomes following major trauma were compared in a regional trauma system and two comparator regions over a 4 year period that spanned the introduction of the trauma system.

Table 2. Distribution of injuries by body region in a UK paediatric major trauma (ISS > 15) population.

Body region	Number (%) of patients ($N = 214$)*
Head/neck	174 (81.3)
Face	2 (0.9)
Chest	40 (18.7)
Abdomen	17 (7.9)
Extremities	52 (24.3)
External	11 (5.1)

* Some patients have injuries in more than one region.
ISS, Injury Severity Score.

A head injury was present in over 80% of paediatric major trauma patients and a severe head injury, Abbreviated Injury Score of 4 or more, was present in 69% of these children. Skeletal trauma to the extremities was the next most common injury followed by injuries to the chest. A smaller number of patients had injuries to the abdominal organs although these injuries account for a larger proportion of immediate management problems. Multiple injuries were present in 30% of these patients. Eighty one (38%) of the 214 paediatric major trauma patients died.

One striking difference between the paediatric trauma population in the USA and other populations, including the UK, is the incidence of penetrating trauma. It is estimated that 10% of paediatric trauma in the USA involves penetrating injuries and that this number is rising in urban areas (Hall et al, 1995). In contrast, in the UK only one case of penetrating injury was recorded in the regional trauma system evaluation (Nicholl et al, 1995) and no cases were recorded in another UK study (Teanby et al, 1993). Similarly, a study in one Australian state found penetrating trauma in only 0.1% of paediatric patients (Cameron et al, 1995). At present therefore, penetrating injuries are relatively rare events in the UK and similar paediatric trauma populations.

Causes of injury

In most trauma populations road traffic accidents are the major cause of injury for both adults and children. In the USA as a whole traffic accidents account for both the largest number of trauma admissions in children and the largest number of trauma deaths (Polhgeers and Ruddy, 1995). In the UK numerous studies have consistently shown road traffic accidents,

J. K. TURNER ET AL

including accidents involving pedestrians and pedal cyclists, to be the predominant cause of injury (Airey and Franks, 1995; Gorman et al, 1995). In the UK 27% of trauma deaths in adults are the result of traffic accidents compared to 50% of paediatric deaths. Falls account for only 4% of deaths in children compared to 29% in adults, again reflecting the problems associated with fractures in the elderly. Drowning, suffocation and foreign body inhalation were more likely causes of death in children (19%: Office for National Statistics, 1996).

Traffic accidents were the most common cause of major trauma to children in the populations studied in the regional trauma centre evaluation (Nicholl et al, 1995), accounting for 63% of all cases, followed by home accidents (14%) and sport and leisure accidents (13%). Falls occurred in 19.6% of these accidents indicating that, although they are the cause of only a small number of deaths in children they make a much larger contribution to the overall trauma workload. Non-accidental injury occurred in less than 5% of paediatric trauma cases in this population.

Volumes

The volume of major trauma that health services have to manage is considerably less in the UK and Australia than in the USA. Table 3 shows the incidence of all major trauma in different regions and the proportion of trauma involving children.

The estimate for the USA reflects regional variations in the incidence of major trauma, but is about three times the incidence in the UK and Australia. The UK studies have estimated that major trauma accounts for approximately 0.08% of all new accident and emergency (A&E) attendance's each year. Less than 10% of these cases will be children. Thus even a large district hospital with 100 000 new attendance's a year would only see between eight and 10 cases of paediatric major trauma a year. One further consideration is when these patients are likely to present to hospital. A detailed analysis of the distribution of time of arrival of major trauma at A&E departments has shown that 88% of paediatric major trauma is admitted to hospital between 0900 and 2100 and 42% in the 4 hours between 1700 and 2100. Only 6.5% of admissions occur in the period midnight to

Table 3. Per capita estimates of major trauma (adults and children) and % involving children.

	USA*	Yorkshire, UK†	Mersey, UK‡	Trauma system evaluation, UK§	Victoria (Australia)¶
Per capita estimate of all major trauma cases/1000	0.5–1	0.27	0.29	0.18	0.25
% involving children (age range in years)	25 (0–18)	10 (0–14)	9.3 (0–15)	8.0 (0–14)	12.0 (0–16)

The per capita estimate from the trauma system data excludes patients who died at the scene. These are included in the other estimates. If it is assumed that the same proportion of deaths at scene occur in this region the per capita rate increases to 0.23/1000.
References: * American College of Surgeons Committee on Trauma, 1993; † Airey and Franks, 1995; ‡ Gorman et al, 1995; § Nicholl et al, 1995; ¶ Cameron et al, 1995.

0900 (Nicholl et al, 1995). This raises questions about whether the same level of service needs to be provided 24 hours a day.

Small numbers and an uneven distribution of demand means that the expected volume of paediatric trauma workload becomes a major consideration along with injury and incident type, when considering possible trauma system designs for the UK. Equally important are the clinical issues pertinent to the management of major trauma. Children differ from adults in their physiological response to injury and consequently have special needs both in terms of how they are managed and who they are managed by.

DIFFERENCES IN MANAGEMENT OF PAEDIATRIC AND ADULT TRAUMA

Children and adults differ with regard to trauma management in two ways. First there are underlying anatomical and physiological differences between adults and children, which also vary at different stages of infancy and childhood. These differences make children even more vulnerable than adults to secondary pathology caused by hypoxia and shock following the traumatic incident. Prompt and effective resuscitation is therefore vital to reduce mortality and limit morbidity.

Second, and partly as a result of this, the effects of trauma on the child differ to that on the adult, leading to notable differences in management particularly with regard to head injury and the management of solid intra-abdominal organ injury.

As we have already discussed, blunt trauma is many times more common in children than penetrating trauma, especially in the UK and head injury predominates. The immediate management of the child head injured patient is similar to that in the adult, that is, prevention of secondary damage by hypoxia, ischaemia and raised intracranial pressure. In adults raised intracranial pressure is almost always largely due to extradural, subdural or intracerebral haemorrhage. The first two of these are amenable to effective treatment by surgical evacuation. However, in children, head injury more often follows a completely different pathology. Cerebral oedema is the main pathology in children (Levin, 1993). It is caused by an increased vascular response to the injury resulting in cerebral hyperaemia, which then progresses to ischaemic oedema when cerebral perfusion falls secondarily to raised intracranial pressure. Currently, treatment is limited to reducing cerebral blood flow by hyperventilation and cerebral oedema by the use of osmotic diuretics. Other treatments such as barbiturate coma, hypothermia and steroids have not been shown to improve outcome. The management of cerebral oedema in a head injured child is one of the major challenges in paediatric trauma.

There are special considerations in infants with head injuries. Severe head injury in infants is significantly associated with child abuse (Hall et al, 1993). The infant's cranial volume can easily increase because of unfused sutures. Therefore large extradural or subdural bleeds or cerebral oedema may occur before neurological signs or symptoms develop. When clinically evident, deterioration is rapid. These infants may show a significant fall in haemoglobin concentration.

Children are vulnerable to solid intra-abdominal organ injuries (liver and spleen). For several years now, non-operable management of such injuries has predominated. In three USA series, 211 children with solid organ injury were described of which 178 (84%) were managed conservatively with no deaths (Pranikoff et al, 1994; Polhgeers and Ruddy, 1995). The treatment criteria for conservative management include a stable circulation and a transfusion requirement of less than half the patient's circulating blood volume (i.e. 40 ml/kg). Even taking into account the risks of blood transfusion (which in fact is no greater with conservative than operative management) there is a clear advantage to patients from this course of management (Velanovich and Tapper, 1993). The overall outcome for patients is a decrease in both immediate mortality and morbidity from operation and in the long-term morbidity and mortality from splenic ablation (Velanovich and Tapper, 1993). The requirements for successful conservative management of solid organ injury in children are careful intravenous fluid management, patient monitoring and the easy availability of a theatre and a paediatric surgeon experienced in this work.

THE ORGANIZATION AND DELIVERY OF TRAUMA SERVICES

Trauma system designs

The aims of any trauma service should be to provide optimal care that gives the highest chance of survival and limits the likelihood of subsequent morbidity. The four essential components of trauma systems are pre-hospital care and transport, acute hospital care, definitive hospital management and rehabilitation.

There are four possible options of trauma system design based on where a trauma patient is taken for treatment:

- Transport to the nearest hospital.
- Transport to the nearest appropriate hospital.
- Transport to a regional trauma centre.
- Transport to a regional paediatric trauma centre.

Each option requires increasingly sophisticated integration of pre-hospital and acute hospital services if the system is to operate efficiently. The first option is the one most commonly adopted in the UK. Patients are taken directly from the scene to the nearest A&E department minimizing the time taken to transport the patient to hospital. The disadvantage of this system is that some of the specialist services trauma patients require, for example neuro or cardiothoracic surgery or paediatric intensive care, may not be available necessitating transfer to other hospitals and therefore delaying definitive care.

In the second option patients are taken to a hospital known to have the specialist facilities an individual patient may require, for example neuro-surgery for a patient with obvious serious head injuries. In the case of children they may be taken directly to a specialist children's hospital. The nearest general hospital may be bypassed and although transport time to hospital may be longer, this could be offset by a reduction in the need for transfer to another hospital. This system is used to a limited extent in the UK, usually in urban areas where there is a choice of hospitals and differences in distance to hospital are relatively small. In such systems, the ambulance service personnel require greater diagnostic and practical skills to limit patient deterioration whilst en route to the emergency department.

The principle of transporting patients to the nearest appropriate hospital is taken one step further in regionalized trauma system designs. Regionalized trauma services have been developed in the USA as a response to the major public health problem that trauma represents there. In particular there was concern that the number of *avoidable* trauma deaths, that is deaths in patients who had survivable injuries that were treatable, was too high. As a result the American College of Surgeons (ACS) Committee on Trauma (1993) have advocated the use of integrated regional trauma systems for the optimal management of major trauma patients. In essence, a regional trauma system comprises a network of hospitals designated as trauma centres at different levels depending on the services available within them. The most seriously injured patients are taken directly to the highest level 1 trauma centre where there is the greatest concentration of specialist services (except in very rural areas where patients may be taken to other centres in the first instance). The ACS guidelines list numerous criteria for the provision of pre-hospital and hospital care. However, the key elements for level 1 trauma centres can be summarized as:

- A 24 hour reception in emergency departments by senior staff.
- All key specialities and services needed for the treatment of trauma on the same site and available (emergency medicine, anaesthetics, general, orthopaedic, neuro, cardiothoracic etc surgery, radiology, laboratory services, operating rooms).
- A high volume of seriously injured patients (about 10–20/week).
- An integrated system with pre-hospital care providers to ensure that seriously injured patients are treated in the trauma centre.

A regional paediatric trauma centre would adopt the same principles but specifically in relation to the management of children (Ramenofsky and Moulton, 1995) and would be expected to care for at least 150 paediatric trauma patients a year.

The rationale for these developments is that the patient receives definitive surgical care as early as possible and that high volumes generate expertise in those caring for patients. As a result mortality, particularly avoidable mortality, and morbidity following trauma should be reduced. Studies have been carried out to measure outcome in different settings and determine whether paediatric trauma is better managed in specialist paediatric or general trauma centres. A summary of the most pertinent of these studies is given in Table 4.

Table 4. Comparative studies of outcome in paediatric trauma patients.

Place	References	Method	Type of patients	Numbers	Conclusions
18 counties in NE New York, USA	Fortune et al, 1992	Retrospective analysis of severely injured children treated by adult trauma surgeons in a paediatric trauma centre	Children ≤15 years with major multiple injuries	303 patients over 4 years	Mortality rate comparable with MTOS norms and other paediatric trauma centres.
New York State, USA	Cooper et al, 1993	Comparison of outcomes in a state with no organized trauma system with outcomes in paediatric trauma centres	Children ≤15 years admitted to hospital with trauma	14 234 state patients 17 099 paediatric trauma registry patients	Survival 10 times greater in paediatric trauma centres for moderately severe brain, skeletal and internal injuries (ISS 15–19). Mortality rates similar for other injuries and comparable severity
Denver, Colorado, USA	Bensard et al, 1994	Paediatric survival in an adult trauma centre compared with young adults and MTOS norms	Patients ≤18 years admitted to level 1 trauma centre	410 ≤15 years 188 16–18 years	No significant differences between observed and expected outcomes
Pennsylvania, USA	Nakayama et al, 1992	Comparison of outcome between paediatric trauma entres, urban non-paediatric centres and rural non-paediatric centres	Patients ≤14 years admitted to 28 trauma centres (TC)	4615 in total 1881 paediatric TC 1293 non-paediatric TC urban 1441 non-paediatric TC rural	Mortality highest in rural trauma centres. Outcome not significantly different in paediatric and urban non-paediatric trauma centres
San Francisco, USA	Knudson et al 1992	Process measures and outcome in paediatric trauma admitted to general level 1 trauma centre compared with MTOS norms	Patients ≤17 years admitted to level 1 trauma centre	353 patients	Outcome comparable with MTOS norms

ISS, Injury Severity Score.

Knudson et al (1992) and Bensard et al (1994) compared the observed outcome of paediatric patients admitted to trauma centres treating patients of all ages with that expected using norms derived from the Major Trauma Outcome Study (MTOS) database. In both studies survival was slightly better than that expected although not significantly so. However both studies included older children (> 14 years) whose management closely approximates that of adults. Outcome in the 14–17 year age group was much better than in younger children in the study by Knudson. In addition the study population also had a high proportion of penetrating trauma (22%) and so cannot be considered representative of the general paediatric trauma population. These studies do show that management of paediatric trauma in adult trauma centres can produce outcomes that are at least as good as those expected when compared to population norms. They cannot demonstrate whether or not outcome is further improved by management at a dedicated paediatric trauma centre. Direct comparison of paediatric and non-paediatric trauma centre care has shown that in the urban environment outcomes are the same (Nakayama et al, 1992). However, the paediatric centre population produced more unexpected survivors. In the same study mortality was higher and there were more unexpected deaths in patients taken to rural non-paediatric centres highlighting the difficulties that arise as a consequence of delays in identifying patients in the field and the need to transport patients over long distances.

All of these studies reflect outcomes in patients managed within well-organized trauma systems. Cooper et al (1993) compared paediatric trauma centre outcomes with those observed in a state with no organized trauma system and found that survival was greatly increased for moderately severe injuries when managed in paediatric trauma centres. However, survival was comparable for other injuries and severity's and patients with severe brain and skeletal injuries appeared to do better in the non-designated hospital. One possible explanation of this anomaly is that the better integration of pre-hospital care in the trauma system resulted in a much larger number of children with unsurvivable injuries arriving at hospital alive. This study was not able to determine whether better outcomes were produced by paediatric trauma centres but did conclude that trauma *systems* save more lives.

There is as yet no definitive evidence that paediatric trauma centres produce substantially better outcomes than general trauma centres. In particular there is a need for more research that concentrates on the younger (< 8 years) moderate to severely injured group who may benefit most. There may of course be benefits from specialized care that have yet to be determined. In particular, outcome in all the published studies has been the relatively crude measure of mortality. Of equal importance is morbidity. It is estimated that 100 000 children under the age of 19 years may become permanently disabled each year as a result of injury (National Safety Council, 1988) but measurement of the physical and emotional conse-quences of trauma has been neglected. Further research in this area is needed to determine whether paediatric centre care results in better out-comes for survivors. However, even if this were to be the case, all of the studies described have recognized the fact that, in reality, all paediatric trauma patients cannot be cared for in paediatric trauma centres. Insufficient numbers of paediatric trauma surgeons and the relatively small proportion of children within the total trauma population means that, outside large urban areas, trauma centres are unlikely to fulfil the requirements for designation as paediatric centres. As a result a large proportion of paediatric trauma will continue to be managed in general trauma centres. The critical factors identified by the present research are that:

- Any trauma centre that cares for paediatric trauma patients should be able to provide services that meet the special needs of this patient group. As the study by Fortune et al (1992) has shown, an adult trauma surgeon with commitment to paediatric care is preferable to a paediatric surgeon with no such commitment.
- A trauma system that allows the early identification of the seriously injured patient and transport to the most appropriate hospital is as important as the trauma centre.

This requires the proper integration of the pre-hospital component of care. In the USA a large proportion of errors identified as contributing to avoidable death have been attributed to this phase of care (Ramenofsky et al, 1984). As a result pre-hospital care has become increasingly sophisticated in two main areas:

- The development of protocols for the field triage of patients that allow the attending ambulance crew to make decisions about where the patient should be transported to. Protocols are based on a combination of physiological measurement (e.g. the Revised Trauma Score), injury type and injury mechanism (Eichelberger et al, 1989; Johnson, 1996).
- The training of ambulance personnel in advanced paediatric life support techniques (Graneto and Soglin, 1993).

The latter is considered particularly important where decisions are made to bypass hospitals and directly transport to a definitive care facility that may entail a longer journey. There is much debate at present about the benefits of advanced life support (ALS) interventions by paramedics in the field and in particular whether, for trauma patients, the strategy should be 'scoop and run' or 'stay and play' (Polhgeers and Ruddy, 1995). What is clear is that if transport times are long then field personnel need to have sufficient skills to maintain vital functions, particularly airway and breathing. At the same time the use of unnecessary procedures should be avoided and, where interventions are needed, they should be performed in transit so that delays are minimized.

In the USA integrated trauma systems based around trauma centres are seen as the way forward in seeking to improve the care given to trauma patients. The next question is, would it be feasible to transfer this model of care to the UK setting?

Do we need trauma centres in the UK?

The preceding discussion has shown that, even in the USA, it is unlikely that care in a specialist paediatric trauma centre can be provided for every child that needs it. This is even less likely in the UK where a trauma centre that would expect to manage the minimum 150 new major trauma patients each year would need to serve a population of at least 6 million people. Apart from a very few closely related large urban areas this means that most centres would have to serve very large geographical areas and hence for many patients the distance to the trauma centre as a primary destination would involve unacceptably long transport times by road. The alternative would be air transport but this would cease to be an option outside daylight hours and patients would then have to go to an alternative, much closer hospital initially and be transferred later. Furthermore, at present, not all ambulance services in the UK could provide paramedics with suitable paediatric ALS skills (Turner and Snooks, 1995).

An alternative would be to transport patients directly to general trauma centres. These would serve smaller geographical areas although, particularly in rural areas, patients at the edge of these areas may still be required to travel long distances. It is also debatable whether such a system would work in the UK. An experimental trauma system in the UK failed to demonstrate any measurable benefits for patients (Nicholl et al, 1995). One of the explanations for this finding was that most of the patients who might have benefited from direct transfer to the trauma centre still went to the nearest hospital. However, improvement in mortality and disability outcomes for seriously injured children will result from attention to all of the links in the 'chain of care'. A 'trauma system' therefore remains a more appropriate concept than a 'trauma centre'. The challenge is to adapt the current network of accident and emergency care into a system that could work.

A possible trauma system for the UK would have the following four aspects:

1. Immediate attention to airway, breathing and in some instances, circulation from paramedics whilst in transit to an initial resuscitation facility. The emphasis of paramedics now should be neither on 'stay and play' nor on 'scoop and run' but on 'move and care'.
2. Full resuscitation and assessment is then provided at the nearest appropriately resourced A&E department. A system of accreditation based on competencies—for example advanced paediatric life support certified staff—could be identified.
3. Selected children, following an agreed triage procedure and as part of a critical care pathway initiated by the paramedic and followed through in the A&E department, would be transferred to a specialist Children's facility that will include paediatric intensive care, neurosurgery, general and genito-urinary surgery, trauma orthopaedics, imaging, family support and preferably also burns and plastics and cardio-thoracic surgery. A transfer service would be provided.
4. Rehabilitation is a long process and should start once the immediate life threat is over to be most successful. Wherever the rehabilitation occurs, it also is better conceived as a rehabilitation system with skills moving at least initially to the child and the family.

In this way an integrated service that delivers the patient to appropriate care could be developed that makes the best use of the current hospital system rather than introducing new facilities that will only cater for the needs of a very small proportion of the population.

CONCLUSIONS

It is well established that trauma is the leading cause of death in children in the UK and similar societies. The multi-factorial causation of trauma and the complex 'chain of care' that the seriously injured child receives means that improvements in outcome are likely to result from incremental change in most components of a trauma system rather than a large change to one resource, however high-profiled.

Despite the pre-eminence of trauma as the foremost cause of death in childhood, fortunately, compared to the adult population, seriously injured children are relatively infrequently brought to a particular institution, and an individual clinician even in a large and busy institution will treat a seriously injured child only occasionally. The implication is that training in trauma management must be repetitive and competency-based to keep skills sharp. In addition the population in the UK is concentrated into large conurbations with a number of more scattered rural areas with much more significant transport problems. It is probable that different solutions for paediatric trauma care may be appropriate for different geographical areas. However these can be based around current services. The UK system of emergency and paediatric care has two particular strengths that are currently growing. A&E medicine is a rapidly developing specialty in which a new faculty has advanced training and in which the concept of consultant-based care has a sound footing. Similarly the specialty of paediatric intensive care has just received recognition and is developing training programmes. There has been a significant increase in public awareness of the ability of paediatric intensive care to contribute to the successful restoration of children to health and well being and a coincident increase in funding. It is these factors that the development of efficient trauma systems can be based on.

Finally, much of the emphasis on trauma care has been aimed at reducing mortality. This is an important but simplistic outcome measure to assess the effectiveness of trauma prevention and treatment systems. Information on morbidity and disability are notably scarce. Without this information, however, only a crude measure of success is available to us. Disability established in childhood clearly has the longest term effect on the child, their family and society, both in terms of lost opportunities and additional burden. It is in this area in particular that future research needs to be concentrated.

REFERENCES

Airey CM & Franks AJ (1995) Major trauma workload within an English Health Region. *Injury* **26:** 25–31.
*American College of Surgeons Committee on Trauma (1993) Planning pediatric trauma care. In *Resources for Optimal Care of the Injured Patient.* Chicago, IL: American College of Surgeons.

*Bensard DD, McIntyre RC, Moore EE et al (1994) A critical analysis of acutely injured children managed in an adult level 1 trauma center. *Journal of Pediatric Surgery* **29:** 11–18.

Cameron P, Dziukas L, Hadj H et al (1995) Major trauma in Australia: a regional analysis. *Journal of Trauma, Injury and Critical Care* **39:** 545–552.

*Cooper A, Barlow D, DiScala C et al (1993) Efficacy of pediatric trauma care: results of a population based study. *Journal of Pediatric Surgery* **28:** 299–303.

DoH (Department of Health) (1991) *The Health of the Nation.* London: HMSO.

Eichelberger MR, Gotschall CS. Sacco WJ et al (1989) A comparison of the Trauma Score, The Revised Trauma Score, and the Pediatric Trauma Score. *Annals of Emergency Medicine* **28:** 425–429.

*Fortune JB, Sanchez J, Graca L et al (1992) A pediatric trauma center without a pediatric surgeon: a four year outcome analysis. *Journal of Trauma* **33:** 130–139.

Gorman DF, Teanby DN, Sinha MP et al (1995) The epidemiology of major injuries in Mersey Region on North Wales. *Injury* **26:** 51–54.

Graneto JW & Soglin DF (1993) Transport and stabilization of the pediatric trauma patient. *Pediatric Clinics in North America* **40:** 365–380.

Hall JR, Reyes HM, Meller JL et al (1993) Traumatic death in urban children, revisited. *American Journal of Diseases in Childhood* **147:** 102–107.

Hall JR, Reyes HM, Meller JL et al (1995) The new epidemic in children: penetrating injuries. *Journal of Trauma* **39:** 487–491.

Johnson WP (1996) Evaluation of the pediatric trauma triage checklist as a prehospital pediatric trauma triage tool for the State of Florida. *Pre-hospital and Disaster Medicine* **11:** 20–26.

*Knudson MM, Shagoury C, Lewis FR (1992) Can adult trauma surgeons care for injured children? *Journal of Trauma* **32:** 729–737.

Levin HS (1993) Head trauma. *Current Opinions in Neurology* **6:** 841–846.

Miller JD, Piper IR & Derden NM (1993) Management of intracranial hypertension in head injury: matching treatment with cause. *Acta Neurologica* **57 (supplement):** S152–S159.

*Nakayama DK, Copes WS, Sacco W (1992) Differences in trauma care among pediatric and non-pediatric trauma centers. *Journal of Pediatric Surgery* **27:** 427–431.

National Safety Council (1988) *Accident Facts.* Chicago, IL: National Safety Council.

*Nicholl JP, Turner J & Dixon S (1995) The cost-effectiveness of the regional trauma system in the North West Midlands. Sheffield: Medical Care Research Unit, University of Sheffield.

Office for National Statistics (1996) *Mortality Statistics 1994.* Series DH2 no.21. London: HMSO.

*Polhgeers A & Ruddy RM (1995) An update on pediatric trauma. *Emergency Medicine Clinics in North America* **13:** 267–289.

Pranikoff T, Schlesinger AE, Polley TZ et al (1994) Resolution of splenic injury after nonoperative management. *Journal of Pediatric Surgery* **29:** 1366–1369.

Ramenofsky ML & Moulton S (1995) The pediatric trauma center. *Seminars in Pediatric Surgery* **4:** 128–134.

Ramenofsky ML, Luterman A, Quindlen E et al (1984) Maximum survival in pediatric trauma: the ideal system. *Journal of Trauma* **24:** 818–823.

Rosenberg HM, Ventura SJ, Maurer JD et al (1996) *Births and Deaths: United States 1995.* Hyatsville, MD: National Centre for Health Statistics.

Teanby DN, Lloyd DA, Gorman DF et al (1993) Paediatric trauma care—the case for centralisation. *Injury* **24:** 275.

Turner J & Snooks H (1995) *England and Wales Ambulance Services: Paramedic Training and Local Policy Survey.* Sheffield: Medical Care Research Unit, University of Sheffield.

Velanovich V & Tapper D (1993) Decision analysis in children with blunt splenic trauma: the effects of observation, splenorrhaphy, or splenectomy on quality-adjusted life expectancy. *Journal of Pediatric Surgery* **28:** 179–185.

8

Severe head injury in children: an audit of the circumstances surrounding the injury and the acute management provided

J. A. EYRE BSc, MBChB, DPhil, FRCP, FRCPH

Professor of Paediatric Neuroscience

PETER W. ROWE MBBS

Senior Registrar in Paediatric Neurology

The Department of Child Health, The Sir James Spence Institute of Child Health, The Royal Victoria Infirmary, Queen Victoria Road, Newcastle upon Tyne NE1 4LP, UK

Head injury is the most important cause of death and long-term morbidity for children over the age of 1 year in the developed world and increasingly recognized to be important also in the developing world. Serious head injuries to children occur most frequently in highly deprived areas. Children tend to be injured as pedestrians in road traffic accidents while playing near their home in the late afternoon or early evening. Unsafe behaviour of children rather than dangerous driving from adults is the most important factor. Strategies implemented in the developed world that have made the environment where children live and play safer, appear to have led to a major reduction in the incidence of fatal head injuries to children.

Audit of the management of children after fatal head injury reveal that 32% had adverse factors in their management that could have been prevented and that probably contributed to their death. The potentially avoidable factors included poor management of airways, failure to diagnose or delayed recognition of intracranial haematomas or serious associated injuries and poor management of transfer between hospital. Twenty two percent of children who died before admission to hospital and 42% of those who died after admission had such potentially avoidable factors. There is some preliminary evidence to suggest that the recent introduction of guidelines for the best management of head injury may be leading to improved care and a reduction in deaths following serious head injury.

Key words: head injury; child; prevention; management.

Head injury is the single most important cause of death in childhood in the developed world (Kraus et al, 1990; Sharples and Eyre, 1994); the mortality rate for example is 5.3/100 000 children per annum in the UK (Sharples et al, 1990b) and as high as 10/100 000 children per annum in the USA

Baillière's Clinical Paediatrics —
Vol. 5, No. 3, August 1997
ISBN 0–7020–2319–1
0963–6714/97/030435 + 16 $12.00/00

(Annegers, 1983; Kraus et al, 1986). It has recently become clear that head injury is also a very significant cause of death and long-term morbidity in the developing world, probably being the third most common cause of death behind infection and diarrhoea (Nordberg, 1994; Forjuoh and Li, 1996; Amakiri et al, 1997).

In all studies the mortality rate from head injury increases with age (e.g. Kraus et al, 1990; Sharples et al, 1990b; Jorgensen, 1995). In the UK, for example, the mortality rate from head injury is 3/100 000 for those aged 1–4 years, 5/100 000 for children aged 5–9 years and 7/100 000 for the age group 10–15 years (Figure 1; Sharples and Eyre, 1994). At all ages the mortality rate from head injury is significantly higher in boys than in girls and the rate of increase with age is also more marked for boys (Hendrick et al, 1963; Jamison and Kaye, 1974; Kraus et al, 1990; Sharples et al, 1990b; Sharples and Eyre, 1993). Thus, by the age of 10–15 years the mortality rate in boys is more than twice that in girls (9.1 *versus* 4.3/100 000; Sharples and Eyre, 1994) and head injury accounts for nearly one third of all deaths in boys in this age group.

Although there have been few population-based studies of morbidity there is no doubt that head injury is also a major cause of acquired neurological disability in childhood. The published rate of admission to hospital in childhood following a head injury varies from approximately 200/100 000 children per annum in the USA (Kalsbeek et al, 1980; Kraus

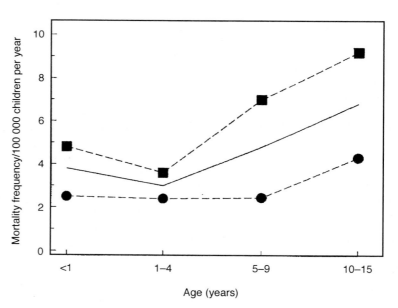

Figure 1. Death in childhood following serious head injury in the Northern Region 1979–1986. Fatality rate by age: in males (■), in females (●) and overall for both sexes (——).

et al, 1984, 1986) to 500/100 000 children per annum in the UK (Sharples et al, 1990b). This variability almost certainly reflects differences in the admission policies between the studies more than differences in the frequency of head injury. There are few studies giving population-based morbidity rates for head injury amongst paediatric admissions but a study in the USA found a rate of 25/100 000 children per annum (Kraus et al, 1986). If these rates are applicable to the UK then 200 children are admitted to hospital every day following a head injury and 25 children are killed or seriously injured.

Head injured children who either die or survive with long-term neuro-psychological handicap are not only tragic figures in their own right but represent a significant financial burden on health, education and social services budgets. In the UK children with head injury occupy 1 000 000 bed days per annum at an annual cost of a least £100 000 000. The Department of Transport estimate the cost to society of a death in childhood is £700 000; the cost of childhood deaths from head injury is thus approximately £420 000 000 per annum. The long-term costs of children who survive severe head injury are likely to amount to more than twice this amount. For both humanitarian and financial reasons it is essential that the highest priority is given both to the prevention of severe head injury to children and to optimizing the management of those who are injured.

It was once thought that little could be done to reduce the mortality and morbidity arising from head injury. Accidents were considered to be unpredictable and thus by their very nature not preventible, and it was thought that traumatic damage to the brain occurred at the time of impact, thus optimizing the subsequent management of the head injured patient was unlikely to improve outcome. It is now abundantly clear that neither assumption is correct. Head injuries are not random events in the population but occur in well defined circumstances. The introduction of appropriate strategies to reduce the risks of head injury to children has the potential, indeed has already been shown, to substantially reduce the incidence and the severity of head injury (e.g. Royal Dutch Touring Club, 1980; Snyder, 1984; Friends of the Earth, 1986; Dorsch et al, 1987). Furthermore, secondary brain injury from hypoxia and cerebral hypo-perfusion in the days following primary traumatic brain injury has now been recognized as a major determinant both of mortality and morbidity after head injury (Graham and Adams, 1971; Reilly et al, 1975; Graham et al, 1978; Jennett and Carlin, 1978; Mendelow et al, 1979; Jeffreys and Jones, 1981; Miller and Becker, 1982; Sharples et al, 1990a) and the prevention of such adverse events has become an important aim of the management of severely head injured patients. This chapter will therefore focus on the audit of two aspects of head injury in childhood; (a) the circumstances in which children receive head injuries and relate these data to strategies for head injury prevention; and (b) the acute manage-ment given to severely injured children to highlight where current management may be failing to prevent secondary brain damage from occurring.

CIRCUMSTANCES IN WHICH CHILDREN SUFFER SERIOUS OR FATAL HEAD INJURIES

The incidence and the mortality rate from serious childhood head injuries is highly correlated with socio-economic deprivation (Preston, 1972; Neresian et al, 1985; Rivara and Barber, 1985; Pless et al, 1987, Sharples et al, 1990b; Jolly et al, 1993). In our population-based study of serious head injury in the Northern Region the rate of fatal head injuries was 15 times greater in the most deprived areas in comparison to the most affluent areas (Figure 2; Sharples et al, 1990b), with nearly 50% of the childhood

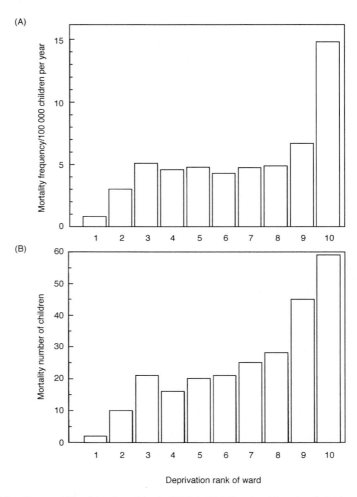

Figure 2. Mortality rate (A) and number of deaths (B) from childhood accidents involving head injury in each of 10 groups of wards in the Northern Region 1979–1986 ranked according to deprivation. 1, the least deprived up to 10, the most deprived (Sharples et al, 1990b).

deaths from head injury occurring in the 20% most deprived wards of the Region (Figure 2B). A similar pattern was found when non-fatal head injuries and serious other traumatic injuries resulting from road traffic were considered, where there was a strong positive relationship between the frequency of such serious accidents and the degree of deprivation (Sharples, 1994).

Serious head injuries do not cluster into black spots but tend to be diffusely scattered, occurring mostly within a very short distance of a child's home (Figure 3A; Sharples et al, 1990b; Ward, 1991, Sharples, 1994). Detailed analysis of the circumstances of serious head injuries reveal that they most frequently occur in unsupervised children playing close to home in the late afternoon and evening (Figure 3B; Jamison and Kaye, 1974; Craft, 1977; Ivan et al, 1983; Kraus et al, 1990; Sharples et al, 1990b; Bannon et al, 1992; Sharples, 1994).

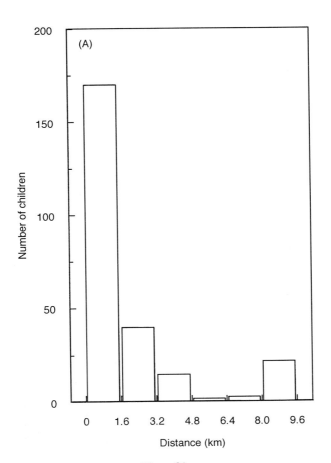

Figure 3A.

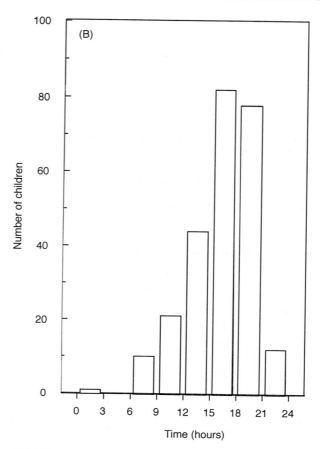

Figure 3 (pages 439–440). Deaths in childhood involving serious head injury in the Northern Region 1979–1986. A, Distance from home to the site of the injury. B, Time of day of the injury (Sharples et al, 1990b).

The analysis of the causes and circumstances of fatal head injuries in the UK reveal that the majority occur following road traffic accidents, where the children are predominantly injured as pedestrians (Figure 4; Illingworth, 1979; Jamison and Kay, 1974; Craft, 1977; Sharples et al, 1990b). These findings contrast with the results of North American and Australian studies, in which the majority of children sustaining fatal head injuries did so as passengers in motor vehicles (Kraus et al, 1990; Simpson et al, 1992; Boswell et al, 1996). Where children have been injured as either pedestrians or cyclists, the incidence of driver negligence is low (Baker et al, 1974b; Rivara and Barber, 1985; Sharples et al, 1990b). The behaviour of children in traffic is often considered unsafe (Russam, 1977; Sandels, 1977; Sharples et al, 1990b).

It has been suggested that such potentially dangerous behaviour can be

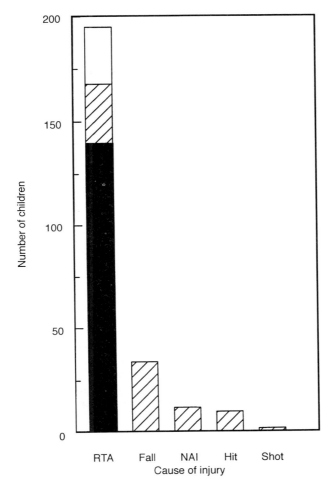

Figure 4. Deaths in childhood involving serious head injury in the Northern Region 1979–1986. Cause of the injury: RTA, road traffic accident; NAI, non-accidental injury; Hit, hit by object (Sharples et al, 1990b). The RTA injuries can be further subdivided into those sustained by pedestrians (▨), cyclists (▧) and car passengers (☐).

modified by education, but the value of road safety education campaigns aimed at children is debated. Children under the age of 12 years have difficulties coping with traffic irrespective of their level of knowledge (Yeaton and Bailey, 1978; Limbourg and Gerber, 1981; Fortenberry and Brown, 1982; Rothengatter, 1984), while children over the age of 12 years possess the maturity to behave properly in traffic but often lack the motivation to do so (Sandels, 1970, 1977).

An alternative strategy has been to aim education programmes at parents, stressing the importance of the supervision of children at play. However, the incidence of serious or fatal accidents is highest in families with large numbers of children (Husband and Hinton, 1972), those headed by a single parent (Wadsworth et al, 1983), families where the mother is mentally or physically ill (Brown and Davidson, 1978) and families where the mothers work outside the home or are caring for a sick relative (Backett and Johnston, 1959). In all these situations the ability of the parent(s) to provide effective supervision is likely to be impaired.

A successful approach to prevention of serious head injuries is the alteration of the environment to make it safer for children. Where such issues have been seriously addressed by Governments and Town Planners there has been a significant reduction in fatal childhood injuries (Snyder, 1984). Such interventions have varied from highly focused measures such as the promotion of child restraints in vehicles and the promotion of cycle helmets, to more general town planning modifications designed to make the areas where children live safer places in which to play. Such schemes have involved appropriate engineering and environmental measures to keep through traffic away from housing estates (Rivara, 1990; Sibert, 1991), traffic calming measures to ensure cars that enter densely populated areas travel at low speeds (Zeeger and Zeeger, 1988) and the provision of playgrounds within a very close distance from children's homes to reduce the numbers of children playing in the street. Although at first sight this may seem an impossibility large task, the observed relationship between the incidence of serious head injury and socio-economic deprivation indicates that selective targeting of measures to those areas of high deprivation would be a cost-effective approach.

There is increasing evidence to suggest that in the last 10 years there has been a consistent and progressive fall in the incidence of severe head injury in children in Europe and Australasia, but perhaps not in the USA (Kraus and Peek, 1995). In the UK nationally there has been a reduction in deaths from trauma injury by 5% per year since 1985 (Office of Population Census and Surveys (OPCS) statistics; Roberts et al, 1996; Roberts and Power, 1996; DiGuiseppi et al, 1997). The greatest reduction has occured in deaths involving road traffic accidents, particularly where children are injured as pedestrians. The ongoing audit of death from head injury in the Northern Region of the UK over the 15 year period 1979–1994, has revealed that the numbers of children dying from head injury has fallen by 50% (Figure 5; our unpublished results). The reduction in deaths, however, has only occured in those dying *before* admission to hospital (Figure 5B), whereas the numbers of children dying after admission to hospital has remained relatively constant (Figure 5C). These data imply that a decrease in severity of the initial injury rather than an improvement in management has led to the reduction in fatalities. The most marked change has been a reduction in the numbers of children receiving fatal head injuries as pedestrians involved in road traffic accidents. This reduction in deaths has coincided with a major campaign by local authorities in the Northern Region to reduce the exposure of children living in housing estates in highly deprived area to road traffic (our unpublished results).

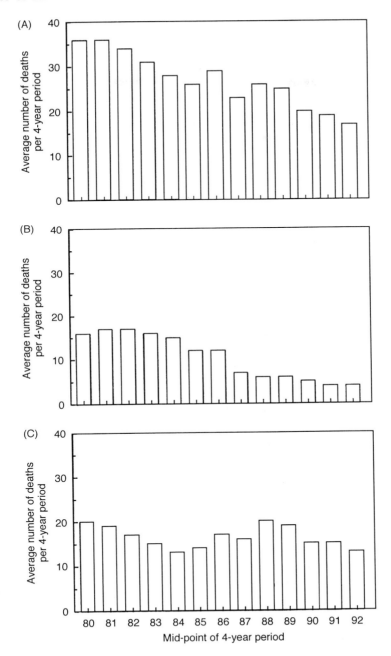

Figure 5. Deaths in childhood involving serious head injury in the Northern Region 1979–1994. Average number of deaths per 4 year period: A, total number of deaths before and after admission to hospital; B, deaths before admission to hospital; C, deaths after admission to hospital.

Roberts et al (1996), have reported a substantial decline in the probability of death over the time period 1989–1995, among children and young adults admitted to hospital with head injury whose Injury Severity Scores (ISS: Baker et al, 1974a) were 16 or greater. The authors concluded that improvement in hospital management was likely to be the primary factor. However, this study did not consider whether there had been a shift in distribution of injury severity towards those with lower ISSs within the range 16–75, and thus explaining a higher probability for survival by a reduction in the severity of the initial injury.

A reduction in death from trauma in childhood has also been reported by Jorgensen (1995) in Denmark in the latter part of his study period (1980–1985). The majority of deaths in this study were a consequence of head injury and the greatest reduction in death rate occured for boys. A recent significant reduction in the incidence of severe head injury has been reported in Australia (Pitt et al, 1994) and over the same time period there has also been a significant reduction in childhood deaths following road traffic accidents (MacKellar, 1995). Finally between 1980 and 1988 there was a significant reduction in serious head injuries in New Zealand including those involving children (Caradocdavies and Dixon, 1995)

The reason for the recent reduction in the incidence of severe head injury in the developed world requires more detailed analysis but it is likely to reflect the multi-dimensional strategies for accident prevention adopted in these countries that have included education, legislation and environmental modification by planning authorities and by parents. Head injury is increasingly recognized as an important public health problem in developing countries. It is unlikely that strategies for the prevention of head injury that have been implemented successfully in the developed world can be simply implemented in the developing world, since the circumstances surrounding injury are likely be different, and the developing world must grapple with limited resources, a higher incidence of deprivation and low levels of education. While extensive research on injury prevention has been conducted in the developed world, such research is still in its infancy in developing countries. Significant resources to allow research directed at preventing unintentional injury in the third world are required if there is to be a world-wide reduction in the incidence of preventable deaths and long-term morbidity from unintentional injuries including severe head injury.

ACUTE MANAGEMENT OF CHILDREN AFTER HEAD INJURY.

Brain damage after head injury arises primarily from direct impact damage and from the pathological, neurometabolic events initiated by the trauma (for a review, see Hovda et al, 1995). At present, despite extensive research, little can be done to ameliorate the primary injury, nor to substantially change the course and outcome of the induced encephalopathy. However, there is considerable evidence that secondary insults to the brain also occur following head injury. The secondary complications include intracranial haematomas where there is a link with an inappropriate delay before evacuation (Mendelow et al, 1979), secondary brain damage caused by hypoxia and hypotension (Graham and Adams, 1971; Miller et al, 1978), uncontrolled convulsions, meningitis and complications from general anaesthesia (Jennett and Carlin, 1978). Studies of the management of adults with severe head injuries indicate that up to 30% have had potentially preventable secondary complications that contribute significantly to mortality and morbidity (Jeffreys and Jones, 1981; Anderson et al, 1988). While these studies included a small number of children, the probability of secondary complications is different in children and the difficulty associated with the assessment of consciousness, particularly of young children, suggests that the incidence of potentially preventible factors in severely head injured children may not simply reflect that observed in adults (Graham et al, 1989; Teasdale et al, 1990). Studies of children dying from multiple injuries, however, indicate that potentially avoidable secondary insults do occur and contribute significantly to death (McKoy and Bell, 1983; Holmes and Reyes, 1984). A population-based study of the incidence of potentially preventible adverse events in the management of children who died after head injury was therefore undertaken in the Northern Region of the UK (Sharples et al, 1990a). The issues of where and by whom the children were managed were also investigated (Sharples et al, 1988), since it has been proposed that the fragmentation of care among different specialities may have been an important factor in the high incidence of sub-optimal care experienced after head injury (Jennett, 1975).

The audit was performed on all children who died after a head injury in the period 1979–1986. The children were identified from the records of the OPCS. The coroner's records, the necropsy reports for all the children and the hospital records of those who were admitted to hospital were reviewed. All children who died at the scene of the accident or who survived the initial injury but had ISSs (Baker et al, 1974a) of 75 were excluded since this score indicates an overwhelming injury with no chance of survival. If a patient with a head injury talks after the injury and dies this has been taken by many to indicate that the primary injury was not overwhelming and that death resulted from secondary complications (Reilly et al, 1975; Jeffreys and Jones, 1981). All such deaths were therefore classified as probably preventable. Other avoidable factors identified in the children were (a) necroscopic evidence of appreciable aspiration of blood or vomit (Yates, 1977); (b) in children who were admitted to hospital a significant intracranial haematoma or (c) life threatening associated injury that was not diagnosed or where treatment was delayed (Jeffreys and Jones, 1981); and (d) episode(s) of unanticipated respiratory arrest after the initial assessment and/or resuscitation in the accident and emergency department (Price and Murray, 1972).

During the 8 year period there were 25 009 hospital admissions aged less than 16 years in the Northern Region for head injury, making head injury the single most important cause for admission to hospital. The children were admitted under the care of a wide range of consultants including paediatricians (53%) general surgeons (14%) orthopaedic surgeons (29%), neurosurgeons (3%) and general physicians (1%). To determine the degree of consensus in the management of head injured children a questionnaire was sent to each of the consultants identified as having cared for children with head injuries. The replies indicated that there was no consensus on such fundamental issues as the indications for skull X-rays, hospital admission, the duration of observation required after admission, the indications for referral to a neurosurgeon and the arrangements made for transfer between hospitals. A similar lack of consensus on the management of head injured adults and children has recently been reported from a review in Canada (Shanon and Feldman, 1994).

During the study period 255 children died from head injury, making head injury the single most important cause of death in those aged more than 1 year. Approximately half of the fatally injured children (125) died before admission to hospital and the remaining 130 died after admission. Thirty-nine children were admitted to, cared for and died at a district general hospital, 68 children were admitted initially at a district hospital and subsequently transferred to a regional neuroscience centre for further management and the remaining 22 fatally injured children were admitted to and cared for only at one of the regional neuroscience centres.

The frequency of avoidable factors in the children who died is summarized in Table 1 (Sharples et al, 1990a). A total of 121 potentially avoidable adverse factors were recorded in 81 (32%) of the 225 children who died; 28 avoidable factors occurred in 27 (22%) of the children who died before admission to hospital and 93 in 54 (42%) of those who died after admission to hospital. Of the potentially avoidable factors occurring after admission, 36 occurred in district general hospitals, 15 during transfer from a district to a regional neurosurgical centre and 42 at a regional neuro-surgical centre.

Twelve children died with head injuries and an undiagnosed major associated injury and in a further child there was considerable delay before diagnosis. These findings are similar to those of the study of deaths from

Table 1. Potentially avoidable factors in the management of children who died after a head injury in the Northern Region 1979–1986.

Died before admission to hospital 125		Died after admission to hospital 130	
Talked and died	3	Talked and died	21
		Delayed or no operation for intracranial haematoma	24
Aspiration	25	Aspiration or respiratory arrest	35
		Delayed or no operation for associated injury	13
Total avoidable factors	28	Total avoidable factors	93
Children with one or more avoidable factors	27 (22%)	Children with one or more avoidable factors	54 (42%)

Source: Sharples et al (1990a).

trauma by the Royal College of Surgeons (Anderson et al, 1988), which concluded that there was a need to improve the initial assessment and management of patients admitted to hospital following multiple trauma.

Of the 68 fatally injured children who were transferred between hospitals in this study, 15 arrived at the referral hospital in a critical condition, 8 in respiratory failure, 7 were severely hypotensive and one was also in status epilepticus. The hazards of interhospital transfer revealed in this study had been highlighted previously (Gentleman and Jennett, 1981, 1990).

There has been considerable discussion concerning the need for routine intubation and ventilation of patients with severe head injury (e.g. Krenn et al, 1975; Miller, 1977; Jennett and Teasdale, 1981; Teasdale and Galbraith, 1981; Turner et al, 1984). The high incidence of respiratory events in this audit and the fact that children in whom such events occurred died with significantly lower ISSs than those without a respiratory complication (Sharples et al, 1990a) supports the argument that intubation and ventilation of severely head injured children should be routine.

Large numbers of children are admitted to hospital for observation following apparently uncomplicated head injuries to enable prompt treatment of potential complications such as intracranial haematomas. It was a matter of concern therefore that 26 children over this time period died with undiagnosed or inadequately treated haematomas.

The high incidence of potentially preventible factors in the management of seriously head injured children highlights the need for the establishment of guidelines for the optimal care of seriously head injured patients, which include the issues specific to the care of children (Sharples and Eyre, 1994)

It is now nearly 20 years since Jennett drew attention to the need for improved management for patients with head injuries (Jennett and Carlin, 1978). Studies in the late 1980s suggested there had been little improvement in the subsequent 10 years (Jeffreys and Jones, 1981; Anderson et al, 1988; Gentleman and Jennett, 1990; Sharples et al, 1990a). There are some early and encouraging indications that there may have been an improvement in the 1990s (Roberts et al, 1996; Graham Grant and Shrouder, 1997). These conclusions are not supported by the preliminary data from the most recent audit of management of fatally head injured children in the Northern Region (Figure 5A and B). The jury is still out and more detailed population-based evaluation is required (our unpublished results).

REFERENCES

Amakiri CNT, Akang EEU, Aghadiuno PU & Odesanmi WO (1997) A prospective study of coroner's autopsies in University College Hospital, Ibadan, Nigeria. *Medicine Science and the Law* **37**: 69–75.

Anderson ID, Woodford M, de Dombal FT & Irving M (1988) Retrospective study of 1000 deaths from injury in England and Wales. *British Medical Journal* **296**: 1305–1308.

Annegers F (1983) The epidemiology of head trauma in children. In Shapeiro I (ed.) *Paediatric Head Trauma*, pp. 1–10. Mount Kisco, NY: Futura Publishing Co.

Backett EM & Johnston AM (1959) Social patterns of road accidents to children: some characteristics of vulnerable families. *British Medical Journal* **i**: 409–413.

Baker SP, O'Neill B Haddon W Jr et al (1974a) A method for describing patients with multiple injuries and evaluating care. *Journal of Trauma* **14**: 187–196.

Baker SP, Robertson LS & Haddon W Jr (1974b) Fatal pedestrian collisions: driver negligence. *American Journal of Public Health* **64**: 318–325.

Bannon MJ, Carter YH & Mason KT (1992) Causes of fatal childhood accidents in North Staffordshire, 1980–1989. *Archives of Emergency Medicine* **9**: 357–366.

Boswell WC, Boyd CR Schaffner D et al (1996) Prevention of pediatric mortality from trauma—are curative measures adequate. *Southern Medical Journal* **182**: 17–23.

Brown GW & Davidson S (1978) Social class, psychiatric disorder of mother, and accidents to children. *Lancet* **i**: 378–380.

Caradocdavies TH & Dixon GS (1995) Hospital morbidity due to head injuries in New Zealand in 1988. *Neuroepidemiology* **14**: 199–208.

Craft AW (1977) A Study of Head Injury in Children. MD Thesis, University of Newcastle upon Tyne.

DiGuiseppi C, Roberts, I & Li L (1997) Influence of changing travel patterns on child death rates from injury: trend analysis. *British Medical Journal* **314**: 710–713.

Dorsch MM, Woodward AJ & Somers RL (1987) Do bicycle safety helmets reduce severity of head injury in real crashes? *Accident Analysis and Prevention* **19**: 183–190.

Forjuoh SN & Li GH (1996) A review of successful transport and home injury interventions to guide developing countries. *Social Science and Medicine* **43**: 1551–1560.

Fortenberry JC & Brown DB (1982) Problem identification, implementation and evaluation of a pedestrian safety programme. *Accident Analysis and Prevention* **14**: 315–322.

Friends of the Earth (1986) The case for safe routes to school: a briefing by Friends of the Earth Road Safety Alert. London: Friends of the Earth.

Gentleman D & Jennett B (1981) Hazards of inter-hospital transfer of comatose head-injured patients. *Lancet* **ii**: 853–855.

Gentleman D & Jennett B (1990) Audit of transfer of unconscious head injured patients to a neuro-surgical unit. *Lancet* **335**: 330–334.

Graham DI & Adams HJ (1971) Ischaemic brain damage in fatal head injuries. *Lancet* **i**: 265–266.

Graham DI, Adams HJ & Doyle D (1978) Ischaemic damage in fatal non-missile head injuries. *Journal of the Neurological Sciences* **39**: 213–234.

Graham DI, Ford I & Hume Adams JH et al (1989) Fatal head injury in children. *Journal of Clinical Pathology* **42**: 18–22.

Graham Grant PT & Shrouder S (1997) Initial assessment and outcomes of head injured patients transferred to a regional neurosurgical service: what do we miss? *Journal of Accident and Emergency Medicine* **14**: 10–12.

Hendrick E, Harwood-Hash D & Hudson A (1963) Head injuries in children: a survey of 4465 - consecutive cases at the hospital for sick children, Toronto, Canada. *Clinical Neurosurgery* **11**: 46–65.

Holmes MJ & Reyes HM (1984) A critical view of pediatric trauma. *Journal of Trauma* **24**: 253–255.

Husband P & Hinton PE (1972) Families of children with repeated accidents. *European Neurology* **8**: 396–400.

Hovda DA, Lee SM, Smith ML et al (1995) The neurochemical and metabolic cascade following brain injury—moving from animal-models to man. *Journal of Neurotrauma* **12**: 903–906.

Illingworth CM (1979) 227 road accidents to children. *Acta Paediatrica Scandinavica* **68**: 869–873.

Ivan L, Choo S & Ventureyra E (1983) Head injuries in children: a 2-year survey. *Canadian Medical Association Journal* **128**: 281–284.

Jamison DL & Kaye HH (1974) Accidental head injury in childhood. *Archives of Disease in Childhood* **49**: 376–381.

Jeffreys RV & Jones JJ (1981) Avoidable factors contributing to the death of head injury patients in Mersey region. *Lancet* **ii**: 459–461.

Jennett B (1975) Who cares for head injuries? *British Medical Journal* **iii**: 267–270.

Jennett B & Carlin C (1978) Preventable mortality and morbidity after head injury. *Injury* **10**: 31–39.

Jennett B & Teasdale G (1981) Management of head injuries in the acute stage. In Jennett B & Teasdale G (eds) *Management of Head Injuries*, pp. 211–251. Philadelphia: FA Davis Company.

Jolly DL, Moller JN & Volkmer RE (1993) The socioeconomic context of child injury in Australia. *Journal of Paediatrics and Child Health* **29**: 438–444.

Jorgensen IM (1995) The epidemiology of fatal unintentional child injuries in Denmark. *Danish Medical Bulletin* **42**: 285–290.

Kalsbeek WD, McLaurin RL, Harris BSH III et al (1980) The National Head and Spinal Cord Injury Survey: major findings. *Journal of Neurosurgery* **53 (supplement):** S19–S31.

Kraus JF & Peek C (1995) The impact of 2 related prevention strategies on head-injury reduction among non fatally injured motor cycle riders, California, 1991–1993. *Journal of Neurotrauma* **12:** 873–881.

Kraus JF, Black M, Hessol M et al (1984) The incidence of acute brain injury and serious impairment in a defined population. *American Journal of Epidemiology* **119:** 186–201.

Kraus JF, Fife D, Cox P et al (1986) Incidence, severity and external cause of pediatric brain injury. *American Journal of Diseases of Children* **140:** 687–693.

Kraus JF, Rock A & Hemyari P (1990) Brain injuries among infants, children, adolescents and young adults. *American Journal of Diseases of Children* **144:** 684–691.

Krenn J, Steinbereithner K, Sporn P, Draxler V & Watzek C (1975) The value of routine respiratory treatment in severe brain trauma. In Penzolz H, Brock M, Hamer J, Klinger M & Spoerri O (eds) *Advances in Neurosurgery*, pp. 134–138. Berlin: Springer Verlag.

Limbourg M & Gerber D (1981) A parent training programme for the road. Safety education of preschool children. *Accident Analysis and Prevention* **13:** 255–267.

Mackellar A (1995) Deaths from injury in childhood in Western Australia, 1983. *Medical Journal of Australia* **162:** 238.

McKoy C & Bell MJ (1983) Preventable traumatic deaths in children. *Journal of Paediatric Surgery* **18:** 505–508.

Mendelow AD, Karmi MZ, Paul KS et al (1979) Extradural haematoma: effect of delayed treatment. *British Medical Journal* **i:** 1240–1242.

Miller JD (1977) The search for optimal management of head injury. *Medical College of Virginia* **13:** 97–106.

Miller JD & Becker DP (1982) Secondary insults to the injured brain. *Journal of the Royal College of Surgeons, Edinburgh* **27:** 292–298.

Miller JD, Sweet RC, Narayan R & Becker DP (1978) Early insults to the injured brain. *Journal of the American Medical Association* **24:** 439–442.

Nersesian WS, Petit M, Shaper R et al (1985) Childhood death and poverty: a study of all childhood deaths in Maine, 1976 to 1980. *Pediatrics* **75:** 41–50.

Nordberg E (1994) Injuries in Africa—a review. *East African Medical Journal* **71:** 339–345.

Pitt WR, Balanda KP & Nixon J (1994) Child injury in Brisbane South 1985–91—implications for future injury surveillance. *Journal of Paediatrics and Child Health* **30:** 114–122.

Pless IB, Verreault R, Arsenault L et al (1987) The epidemiology of road accidents in childhood. *American Journal of Public Health* **77:** 358–360.

Preston B (1972) Statistical analysis of child pedestrian accidents in Manchester and Salford. *Accident Analysis and Prevention* **4:** 323–332.

Price DJE & Murray A (1972) The influence of hypoxia and hypotension on recovery from head injury. *Injury* **3:** 218–223.

Reilly PL, Graham DI, Adams JH & Jennett B (1975) Patients with head injury who talk and die. *Lancet* **ii:** 375–377.

Rivara FP (1990) Child pedestrian injuries in the United States. Current status of the problem, potential interventions, and future research needs. *American Journal of Diseases of Childhood* **144:** 692–696.

Rivara FP & Barber M (1985) Demographic analysis of childhood pedestrian injuries. *Pediatrics* **76:** 375–381.

Roberts I & Power C (1996) Does the decline in child injury mortality vary by social class? A comparison of class specific mortality in 1981 and 1991. *British Medical Journal* **313:** 784–786.

Roberts I, Cambell F, Hollis S & Yates D (1996) Reducing accident death rates in children and young adults—the contribution of hospital care. *British Medical Journal* **313:** 1239–1241.

Rothengatter T (1984) A behavioural approach to improving the traffic behaviour of young children. *Ergonomics* **27:** 147.

Royal Dutch Touring Club (1980) *Woonerf*. The Hague: Royal Dutch Touring Club.

Russam K (1977) The psychology of children in traffic. In Jackson RH (ed.) *Children, the Environment and Accidents*, pp 49–65. Tunbridge Wells: Pitman Medical.

Sandels S (1970) Young children and traffic. *British Journal of Educational Psychology* **40:** 111–115.

Sandels S (1977) An overall view of children in traffic. In Jackson RH (ed.) *Children, the Environment and Accidents*, pp 20–27. Tunbridge Wells: Pitman Medical.

Shanon A & Feldman W (1994) Management of moderate head injury in childhood: degree of consensus among Canadian pediatric emergency physicians. *Pediatric Emergency Care* **10:** 322–325.

Sharples PM (1994) *Preventing mortality and morbidity from head injury in childhood*. PhD thesis, University of Newcastle, UK.

Sharples PM & Eyre JA (1994) Head injury in childhood: the most important cause of death and acquired handicap. *Current Paediatrics* **3:** 225–229.

Sharples PM, Aynsley-Green A & Eyre JA (1988) Management of children with head injuries in district general hospitals. *Archives of Disease in Childhood* **63:** 570.

Sharples PM, Storey A, Aynsley-Green A & Eyre JA (1990a) Avoidable factors contributing to death of children with head injury. *British Medical Journal* **300:** 87–91.

Sharples PM, Storey A, Aynsley-Green A & Eyre JA (1990b) Causes of fatal childhood accidents involving head injury in Northern region, 1979–86. *British Medical Journal* **301:** 1193–1197.

Sibert JR (1991) Accidents to children: the doctor's role. Educational or environmental change? *Archives of Disease in Childhood* **66:** 890–893.

Simpson DA, Blumbergs PC, Mclean AJ & Scott G (1992) Head injuries in infants and children—measures to reduce mortality and morbidity in road accidents. *World Journal of Surgery* **16:** 403–409.

Snyder MB (1984) Regulations for pedestrian and cycle safety: why, who, what and how to regulate. In *Metropolitan Association of Urban Designers and Environmental Planners, Proceedings of the Seminar of Bicycle/Pedestrian Planning and Design*, pp 553–564. Florida and New York: American Society of Civil Engineers.

Teasdale G & Galbraith H (1981) Head trauma and intracranial haemorrhage. In Grenik A & Safar P (eds) *Brain Failure and Resuscitation*, pp 185–219. Edinburgh: Churchill Livingstone.

Teasdale GA, Murray G, Anderson E et al (1990) Risks of acute traumatic intracranial haematoma in children and adults: implications for managing head injuries. *British Medical Journal* **300:** 363–367.

Turner E, Hilfiker O, Braun U et al (1984) Metabolic and hemodynamic response to hyperventilation in patients with head injuries. *Intensive Care Medicine* **10:** 127–132.

Wadsworth J, Burnell J, Taylor B & Butler N (1983) Family type and accidents in preschool children. *Journal of Epidemiology and Community Health* **37:** 100–104.

Ward H (1991) *Preventing road traffic accidents to children—the role of the NHS*. London: Health Education Authority.

Yates D (1977) Airway patency in fatal accidents. *British Medical Journal* **ii:** 1249–1251.

Yeaton WH & Bailey JS (1978) Teaching pedestrian safety skills to young children; an analysis and one year follow up. *Journal of Applied Behaviour Analysis* **11:** 315–329.

Zegeer CV & Zeeger SF (1988) Designing and safer walking environment. *Traffic Safety* **88:** 16–19.

9

Why have injury death rates fallen?

IAN ROBERTS MBChB, MRCP, PhD

Senior Lecturer in Epidemiology and Director, Child Health Monitoring Unit
Institute of Child Health, 30 Guilford Street, London WC1N 1EH, UK

DAVID W. YATES MD, MCh, FRCS, FFAEM

Professor of Emergency Medicine, University of Manchester and Honorary Consultant, Hope Hospital
Department of Accident and Emergency Medicine, University of Manchester, Hope Hospital, Salford M67 8HD, UK

Injury is the leading cause of death in children and adolescents. Over the past two decades injury death rates in childhood have fallen steadily. This decline is often presumed to be the result of injury prevention activities. But is this supported by the available research evidence? In this chapter a number of potential explanations for the decline in injury death rates are explored. Part of the fall in childhood injury mortality can be explained by trends in children's travel patterns, such that fewer children nowadays walk or cycle. Evidence from the Major Trauma Outcome Study and from police accident records show that there has also been a substantial decline in injury case-fatality—the proportion of people who die at any given level of injury severity. The steep decline in injury case-fatality underscores the public health importance of high quality trauma care systems. An efficient system for the transport and acute care of seriously injured children and young adults must be an integral part of any public health strategy to reduce injury death rates.

Key words: unintentional injury; pedestrian; cyclist; injury prevention; case-fatality; trauma care.

Injury is a leading cause of death in children and young adults. Not surprisingly, many countries have placed the reduction of child injury death rates high on the public health agenda. As a result, there has been a burgeoning of interest in injury prevention. For example, in England, a national target was set to reduce the injury death rate among children under 15 by at least 33% by the year 2005 (DoH, 1992). At the same time, a government task force on accident prevention was established to ensure that preventive activity was properly informed and co-ordinated. So far, progress towards the target has been encouraging. Between 1985 and 1992, the child injury death rate declined by 34% to 5.4 deaths/100 000 children in 1992 (DiGuiseppi et al, 1997). Indeed, if present trends continue, the target will almost certainly be exceeded. Declines of a similar magnitude have been observed over the same period for children aged 0–19 years in the USA, and for Western Australian children aged 0–14. But does this necessarily represent a success for injury prevention?

In England and Wales, motor vehicle traffic accidents involving children as pedestrians, vehicle occupants and cyclists, comprise about half of all injury deaths. Pedestrian accidents alone make up 32% of injury deaths (DiGuiseppi et al, 1996). For many years, pedestrian death rates have fallen, in line with total injury mortality (Roberts, 1993). Between 1985 and 1992, the child pedestrian death rate in England and Wales fell by 37%.

Some of the decline can be explained by the reduction in children's independent travel. For example, Hillman found that in 1971, 80% of 7 and 8 year old English children were allowed to walk to school without adult supervision, but in 1990 the corresponding figure was only 9% (Hillman et al, 1991). There has also been a considerable decline in children's walking and cycling. Data from the Department of Transport's (DoT) National Travel Surveys show that between 1985 and 1992 the annual average number of miles walked by children declined by 20%, from 247 miles to 198 miles/child per year, and the annual average number of miles cycled fell by 26% from 38 miles to 28 miles per year. (DoT, 1995). Nevertheless, even when the denominator of the death rates is miles walked, there is still evidence of a substantial decline. Poisson regression modelling using death certificate data and data from the National Travel Surveys shows that pedestrian traffic deaths/mile walked have declined by 24% and cycling death/mile by 20% (DiGuiseppi and Roberts, 1996).

An alternative explanation for the decline in injury death rates could be the effect of prevention programmes. For example, the reduction in child pedestrian mortality may be due to pedestrian injury prevention programmes such as the Green Cross Code. However, there is very little evidence in support of this explanation. In Britain, as in most developed countries, the main thrust of preventive effort has been pedestrian education (Roberts, 1993). However, data from rigorous evaluation studies shows that these programmes are of limited value. For example, Rivara et al (1991) evaluated a community-wide programme to train school children in street-crossing skills. Children's street crossing was observed pre-training and post-training and was graded on four safety related behaviours: walking on the kerb, stopping at the kerb, looking before crossing and looking whilst crossing. Training did not improve performance on the first two behaviours, although there was an increase in looking. Even if the limited behavioural gains of this pedestrian education project were maintained over time, there is no evidence that they would result in reduced injury rates. A comprehensive overview of pedestrian education programmes carried out by the Organization for Economic Co-operation and Development (OECD) also concluded that there was little evidence to support the effectiveness of pedestrian education programmes in reducing injury rates (OECD, 1983). It would appear implausible therefore that pedestrian injury prevention programmes alone account for the declining death rates.

If the decline in death rates cannot be explained by changes in children's exposure to risk, nor to the effect of prevention programmes, might it not be due to better hospital care of injured children, such that fewer injured children die? If this were shown to be a possibility then it would underscore the importance of collecting data that would allow the extent of the decline in case-fatality to be properly quantified. It would also suggest a radical review of the prioritization of public health and clinical strategies for injury control. This chapter will review the evidence for a decline in the injury case-fatality rate.

HAS THERE BEEN A DECLINE IN INJURY CASE-FATALITY?

Evidence from police accident records

Case-fatality is defined as the cumulative incidence of death among those who have the health problem of interest. In the case of accidental injury, a number of data sources are available that provide an indication of whether there has been a change in the probability of death after injury. For example, DoT data, based on police reports show that over the past two decades, the number of police reported child pedestrian casualties fell by 49%, whereas the number of deaths fell by 61% (DoT, unpublished data). In other words, the decline in deaths is proportionately larger than the decline in casualties, suggesting that there has been a decline in the pedestrian injury case-fatality rate. However, these data must be viewed with caution. First, child pedestrian injuries are significantly under-reported in police accident databases and changes over time in casualty numbers might simply reflect changes in the extent of under-reporting (Mass and Harris, 1984). Second, very young children have a higher case-fatality rate, in which case the apparent overall reduction in case-fatality could simply be due to a change in age distribution of injured children, with younger children now making up a smaller proportion of the total casualties. Furthermore, even if these data were valid, it would be impossible to determine whether the decline in mortality was due to improvements in medical care or a decrease in injury severity. Without an objective measure of severity, a decline in the proportion of injured patients who die may simply reflect the inclusion in the casualty statistics of less severely injured children. Clearly, in order to assess whether hospital case-fatality has changed, it is necessary to control very carefully for changes in injury severity.

Controlling for injury severity

A pre-requisite for the valid estimation of temporal trends in injury case-fatality is the ability to control for changes in injury severity. Ideally, trends in case-fatality would be examined in patients who have exactly the same pattern of injuries of identical severity. Unfortunately, this is not possible in practice, but the general aim of comparing patients of similar injury severity can be achieved by the use of objective injury severity scoring systems (Yates, 1990). For example, a study in Leeds compared 186 cases of major trauma (children and adults) admitted to two hospitals in Leeds in 1988/89, with 198 cases admitted in 1992/93 (Burdett-Smith et al, 1995). Injury Severity Score (ISS), age and sex distribution were similar for the two groups. In the earlier period, 48% of the patients died as a result of their injuries, compared with 24% in the latter period. The investigators estimated that for every 100 patients treated in 1992/93, 25 lives were saved compared with 1988/89. The results of this study are therefore consistent with observations made on the basis of police accident data, in showing a substantial reduction in the injury case-fatality rate. Nevertheless, there are some potential methodological problems with this study that deserve consideration. Although case-fatality was compared for two groups of patients with broadly similar ISSs, the possibility that there were subtle differences in injury severity, or other differences in predictors of injury outcome remains. Furthermore, the Leeds study compared prospectively collected data for the later period, with a retrospective case series for the earlier period, and bias may have been introduced as a result of differences in data collection. Both these problems however, were addressed in a more recent study of injury case-fatality among children and young adults admitted to hospitals participating in the Major Trauma Outcome Study (MTOS)

Evidence from the MTOS

Probably the most compelling evidence for a reduction in injury case-fatality is provided by an analysis of data from the UK MTOS. This is a multi-centre prospective cohort study designed to assess the effectiveness of the management of serious injury in the UK (Yates et al, 1992). Information is collected on all seriously injured patients who are admitted to participating hospitals for more than 3 days, or die from their injuries, or are transferred to or from another hospital, or are admitted to intensive care. For each patient a complete list of injuries is used to generate an ISS, and recordings of the respiratory rate, systolic blood pressure and Glasgow coma scale are used to calculate a Revised Trauma Score (RTS: Baker et al, 1974, Baker and O'Neill, 1976; Champion et al, 1987). The use of objective injury scoring allows an examination of trends in the probability of death un-confounded by injury severity.

Roberts et al (1996) used data from the MTOS to assess the extent to which injury case-fatality has fallen. In this study, case-fatality was defined as the proportion of patients with an ISS of 16 or more who died as a result of their injuries. An ISS of 16 or more is conventionally taken to represent major trauma. Trends in case-fatality were examined over the 7 year period from 1989 to 1995. Because the method of wounding (blunt or penetrating) has an independent effect on the probability of death, and may have changed over time, analyses were restricted to patients with blunt trauma. Penetrating trauma accounts for a small proportion (5%) of severe trauma.

Logistic regression modelling was used to examine temporal trends in the probability of death, controlling for age, ISS and RTS. Expected mortality was calculated as the sum of the predicted probabilities of death for each individual.

Over the 7 year study period, a total of 16 710 injured people aged 0–24 years fulfilled the inclusion criteria of the MTOS. Of these 3394 (20%) had an ISS of 16 or more. Of the patients with blunt trauma, 2290 (71%) had been involved in a road traffic accident, and 531 (17%) had been injured in a fall. The distribution of these and other causes of injury were similar from year to year. There was no change in the median Injury Severity Score over time. The median Injury Severity Score was 25 in every year. The annual decline in the observed mortality of patients with an ISS of 16 or more is shown in Table 1. In each age group there is clear evidence for a decline in the probability of death. When expected mortality was calculated using logistic regression based on ISS and RTS, the ratio of observed to expected deaths showed a similar decline (Table 1). The log odds of death shows an almost linear decline across the 7 year period in all 3 age groups (Figure 1).

Table 2 gives the odds ratios for average yearly trend in each age group adjusted for ISS and RTS. For all age groups, there was a significant decline in the probability of death. Modelling the trend using age group as a confounding variable and controlling for RTS and ISS, the overall odds ratio for the yearly trend was 0.84 (95% confidence interval 0.79–0.89). Figure 2 shows the decline in the estimated odds of death in each year calculated relative to the baseline year of 1989, controlling for ISS, RTS

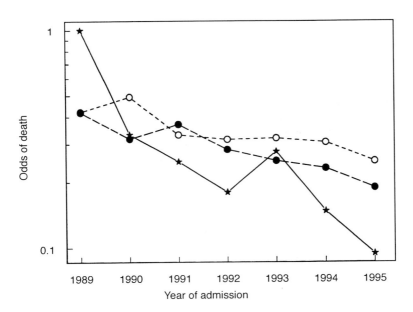

Figure 1. Log odds of death in each year of admission for three age groups. ($\star$), 0–4 years; ($\bullet$), 5–14 years; (O), 15–24 years.

Table 1. Trends in case-fatality and comparison with expected mortality rates for children and young people, 1989–1995 (Injury Severity Score ≥ 16).

Year	0–4 years				5–14 years				15–24 years			
	Total cases	Observed mortality (%)	Expected mortality (%)	Observed/ expected ratio	Total cases	Observed mortality (%)	Expected mortality (%)	Observed/ expected ratio	Total cases	Observed mortality (%)	Expected mortality (%)	Observed/ expected ratio
1989	6	50.0	36.5	1.37	44	29.5	20.4	1.45	155	29.7	20.4	1.46
1990	16	25.0	21.3	1.17	58	24.1	22.6	1.07	145	33.1	24.9	1.33
1991	70	20.0	18.3	1.09	129	27.1	24.4	1.11	284	25.0	23.7	1.05
1992	52	15.4	13.8	1.11	135	22.2	22.0	1.01	356	24.2	24.1	1.00
1993	41	22.0	14.0	1.56	128	20.3	18.6	1.09	310	24.5	26.8	0.92
1994	84	13.1	18.2	0.72	240	19.2	22.0	0.87	500	23.8	27.5	0.87
1995	34	8.8	15.7	0.56	154	16.2	19.0	0.85	289	20.4	22.2	0.92

Table 2. Odds ratio for average yearly trend in each age group adjusted for Injury Severity Score and Revised Trauma Score.

Age (years)	All hospitals OR (95% CI)	Original cohort of hospitals OR (95% CI)
0–4	0.79 (0.63, 0.99)	0.88 (0.65, 1.20)
5–14	0.87 (0.78, 0.97)	0.88 (0.76, 1.01)
15–24	0.83 (0.77, 0.90)	0.80 (0.72, 0.87)

OR, odds ratio; CI, confidence interval.

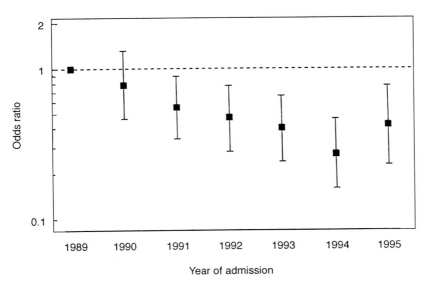

Figure 2. Estimated odds of death with 95% confidence intervals adjusted for Injury Severity Score, Revised Trauma Score and age for each year of admission relative to the baseline year of 1989.

and age. Since 1989 there has been a clear downward trend in the odds of death that can not be explained by differences in severity of injury or age.

CONCLUSION

There has been a substantial decline in hospital case-fatality rate among children and young adults admitted for the treatment of severe injury. Data from the MTOS show that after controlling for injury severity, there has been an annual decline in the odds of death in hospital of 21% for children under the age of 5, 13% for children aged 5–14 years, and 17% for people aged 15–24 (Roberts et al, 1996). These results suggest that reductions in hospital case-fatality have made an important contribution to reaching the Health of the Nation targets in England.

The validity of this conclusion, based on the methodology of the MTOS, merits careful examination. The severity of injury is a major determinant of outcome so the ability to adequately control for injury severity is essential. This is turn depends on the accuracy of the measurement of injury severity. Misclassification may result from deficiencies in the scoring systems themselves or from substantial inter-rater variation in the scoring of individual patients (Zoltie and de Dombal, 1993). Severity scoring for the MTOS is only carried out by trained staff at the North Western Injury Research Centre but misclassification may have arisen because of variability in the accuracy of recording of injury from the case-notes. Bias might also have arisen if there has been a change in recruitment criteria during the study period. Whilst the use of unambiguous inclusion criteria would be expected to minimize this, the extent to which subjective bias accounts for the decline in case-fatality remains a matter for judgement.

This conclusion that there has been a decline in injury case-fatality in children is consistent with police accident data, and the study in Leeds (Burdett-Smith et al, 1995) but the reasons for the decline are open to speculation. Over the past decade there have been considerable changes in the care of the seriously injured patient in the UK. For example, the Royal College of Surgeons report on 1000 trauma deaths in 1988 stimulated the introduction of Advanced Trauma Life Support (ATLS) courses in many centres in the UK (Anderson et al, 1988; Skinner, 1993). There has also been a burgeoning of interest in the concept of the rapid multi-disciplinary team approach to resuscitation. It is possible therefore that the observed improvement in survival in recent years is due to better initial assessment and resuscitation in hospital and the provision of integrated management from the scene of the incident through to intensive care and definitive surgery. There was certainly the potential for a reduction in the hospital case-fatality rate. For example, Sharples examined the prevalence of avoidable complications contributing to the death of children with head injuries in Newcastle from 1979 to 1986 (Sharples et al, 1990). For children who died in hospital, there was a high prevalence of potentially avoidable factors, including delayed diagnosis of intra-cranial haemorrhage and intra-abdominal injury, inadequate airway management and poor management of inter-hospital transfers.

Whatever the reason, the observed decline in hospital case-fatality highlights the importance of medical care in reducing injury death rates among children and young adults. Although the medical historian Thomas McKeown has argued that medical care has played a relatively minor role in the reduction of population death rates, the evidence reviewed in this chapter suggests that injury mortality may be an important exception. This conclusion is supported by recent ecological evidence showing that increased Gross National Product per capita and increased proportional spending on health care is associated with decreasing case-fatality rates among traffic accident victims (Soderlund and Zwi, 1995). An efficient system for the transport and acute care of seriously injured children and young adults should be an integral part of any public health strategy to reduce injury death rates.

Although the evidence reviewed in this chapter supports the conclusion that the care of patients with multiple injuries is improving in the UK, it should be emphasized that case-fatality is a relatively crude measure of the outcome of trauma care. A measure of the extent of disability among those who survive is also required. Bearing in mind the steep decline in injury death rates, future research efforts should aim to secure a deeper understanding of the distribution and determinants of injury related disability. The prevention of injury related disability is a worthy goal for both preventative and curative services.

REFERENCES

Anderson ID, Woodford M, DeDombal FT & Irving M (1988) Prospective study of 1000 deaths from injury in England and Wales. *British Medical Journal* **296**: 1305–1308.

Baker SP & O'Neill B. (1976) The injury severity score: an update. *Journal of Trauma* **16**: 882–885.

Baker SP, O'Neill B, Haddon W & Long, WB (1974) The injury severity score: a method for describing patients with multiple injuries and evaluating emergency care. *Journal of Trauma* **14**: 187–196.

Burdett-Smith P, Airey M & Franks A (1995) Improvements in trauma survival in Leeds. *Injury* **26**: 455–458.

Champion HR, Copes WS, Gann DS, Gennarelli TA & Flanagan ME (1987) A revision of the trauma score. *Journal of Trauma* **27**: 370–378.

DoH (Department of Health). (1992) *The Health of the Nation.* London: HMSO.

DoH (Department of Health) (1995) *Fit for the Future: Second Progress Report on the Health of the Nation.* London: HMSO.

DoT (Department of Transport) (1995) *Transport Statistics Report: National Travel Survey 1992–94.* London: HMSO.

DiGuiseppi C, Roberts I & Li L (1997) Influence of changing travel patterns on child injury death rates. *British Medical Journal* (in Press).

Hillman M, Adams J & Whitelegg J (1991) *One False Move: A Study of Children's Independent Mobility.* London: Policy Studies Institute.

Mass MW & Harris S (1984) Police reporting of road accident inpatients. *Accident Analysis and Prevention* **16**: 167–184.

OECD (Organization for Economic Co-operation and Development.) (1983) *Traffic Safety of Children.* Paris: OECD.

Rivara FP, Booth CL, Bergman AB, Rogers LW & Weiss J (1991). Prevention of pedestrian injuries to children: effectiveness of a school training program. *Paediatrics* **88**: 770–775.

Roberts I (1993) Why have child pedestrian death rates fallen? *British Medical Journal* **306**: 1737–1739.

Roberts I, Hollis S, Campbell F, & Yates D (1996) Reducing death rates in children and young adults: the contribution of hospital care. *British Medical Journal* **13**: 1239–1241.

Sharples PM, Storey A, Aynsley-Green A & Eyre J (1990) Avoidable factors contributing to death of children with head injury. *British Medical Journal* **301**: 1193–1197.

Skinner DV (1993). Advanced trauma life support. *Injury* **24**: 147–149.

Soderlund N & Zwi AB (1995) Traffic-related mortality in industrialised and less developed countries. *Bulletin of the World Health Organisation* **73**: 175–182.

Yates DW (1990). Scoring systems for trauma. *British Medical Journal* **301**: 1090–1094.

Yates DW, Woodford M & Hollis S (1992) Preliminary analysis of the care of injured patients in 33 British hospitals: first report of the United Kingdom major trauma outcome study. *British Medical Journal* **305**: 737–740.

Zoltie N, de Dombal FT (on behalf of the Yorkshire Trauma Audit Group) (1993) The hit and miss of ISS and TRISS. *British Medical Journal* **307**: 906–909.

10

The management of burns and scalds

J. C. LAWRENCE PhD, CBiol, FIBiol

Senior Research Fellow
Wound Healing Research Unit, Llandough Hospital, Penlan Road, Llandough, South Glamorgan CF64 2XX, UK

CAROLYN A. REID MBBS, FRCS(C)

Consultant Plastic Surgeon
Royal Victoria Infirmary & Associated Hospitals NHS Trust, Queen Victoria Road, Newcastle upon Tyne NE1 4LP, UK

The practical management of the paediatric burn is outlined including first aid and resuscitation, dressings and wound care. In order to give a perspective to the problem, the causation, epidemiology, bacteriology, control of infection and wound healing are discussed.

Key words: burns; accident; epidemiology; bacteriology; infection; wound healing; assessment of burn; toxic shock syndrome; dressings; skin substitutes.

EPIDEMIOLOGY

Burns, in the context used here, includes all thermal injuries other than those attributable to water, steam and aqueous solutions except those containing corrosive substances. There is a paucity of national epidemiological data, apart from deaths which are reported annually (OPCS, 1991, 1992, 1993, 1995a,b,c), and limited information from the Home Accident Surveillance System Annual Reports. The data in this Chapter derives from published information on cases received at Birmingham Accident Hospital in the 1980s (Lawrence, 1991a, 1995, 1996a).

Children aged under 15 years comprised 45% of the 4163 burn and scald admissions; 1473 of the 1885 children were below school age (Table 1). As might be expected, children aged between 1 and 2 years of age suffer most burns and scalds as they develop mobility and explore their environment but lack the experience to recognize hazards (Lawrence, 1991a). Boys are more susceptible than girls and scalds considerably outnumber burns (Table 1). However, by the time a child enters school the risk of thermal injury differs little from that of adults of working age (Lawrence, 1991a, 1996a).

Baillière's Clinical Paediatrics—
Vol. 5, No. 3, August 1997
ISBN 0–7020–2319–1
0963–6714/97/030461 + 18 $12.00/00

Table 1. Numbers of burned or scalded children admitted to the West Midlands Regional Burns Unit from 1 January 1980 to 31 December 1989.

	<5			5–14			All children		
Age (years)	M	F	P	M	F	P	M	F	P
Population (thousands)	173	164	347	355	334	689	528	498	1026
Burns	183	133	316	182	56	238	365	189	554
Deaths	1	4	5	6	1	7	7	5	12
Incidence per 10K population	10.6	8.1	9.1	5.1	1.7	3.5	6.9	3.8	5
Scalds	692	465	1157	87	87	174	779	552	1331
Incidence per 10K population	40.0	28.4	33.3	2.5	2.6	2.5	14.7	11.1	12
All burns and scalds	875	598	1473	269	143	412	1144	741	1885
All deaths	1	4	5	6	1	7	7	5	12

It is gratifying to note that the proportion of children admitted to the burns unit has almost halved compared with 40 years ago (Lawrence, 1995). A cautious national estimate suggested about 13 000 burns and scalds admissions occur annually (Lawrence, 1996a), and childhood admissions could be over 5000.

MORTALITY

Case mortality in the series of Birmingham data was 0.6% and all deaths were associated with burns, whereas case mortality for all admissions (i.e. including adults) was 5.9%. The probability of death increases with extent of burn and age of the victim, thus children have a better prognosis than adults for burns up to 35% of total body surface area (Lawrence, 1995). However, it has been suggested that the very young have a worse prognosis (Roi et al, 1981). Mortality charts for retrospective assessment of results are available (Bull, 1971; Lawrence, 1991b, 1995) and prognosis in burns was recently reviewed (Barrett, 1996).

CAUSES OF BURNS

The prime causes of burns are shown in Table 2. Space heating, contact with hot objects and spilt fat are common causes in young children, whereas outside fires, flammable liquids and electricity are common in older male children. Six deaths were associated with the latter two causes, most of the other deaths resulted from house fires. Burn severity is often worsened if the victim is trapped or rendered unconscious and deep, extensive burns frequently ensue if clothing catches fire; a high mortality rate is associated with such cases (Lawrence, 1995). Numbers of burns and deaths due to space heating have declined over the last 40 years, whereas those caused by flammable liquid have markedly increased (Lawrence, 1995). Legislation, together with changes in fashion and composition of fabrics, have contributed to the decline in nightwear burns but these may have increased in recent years (Lawrence and Gowar, 1993).

Table 2. Prime causes of burns to children admitted to the West Midlands Regional Burns Unit from January 1980 to December 1989.

Age (years)	<5			5–14			All children		
	M	F	P	M	F	P	M	P	P
Space heating	48	38	86	9	6	15	57	44	101
		(1)							
Cooking stoves	5	6	11	3	11	14	8	17	25
Spilt fat	28	15	43	11	5	16	39	20	59
Hot objects	33	24	57	3	4	7	36	28	64
House fires	20	10	30	3	4	7	23	14	37
	(1)	(3)	(4)		(1)		(1)	(4)	(5)
Outside fires	2	0	2	34	8	42	36	8	44
Electricity	7	3	10	23	3	26	30	6	36
				(3)			(3)		(3)
Flammable liquid	5	13	18	53	10	63	58	23	81
				(3)			(3)		(3)
Other and unknown	35	24	59	43	5	48	78	29	107
	(1)		(1)	(1)		(1)	(2)		(2)
All burns	183	133	316	182	56	238	365	189	554
	(1)	(4)	(5)	(6)	(1)	(7)	(7)	(5)	(12)

Deaths are in parentheses (no entry if zero).

CAUSES OF SCALDS

The prime causes of scalding are shown in Table 3. Kettles, especially electric kettles, are a particularly common cause and the problem has been reviewed (Lawrence and Cason, 1994). Bathing is another particularly common cause, as are mishaps with tea. The very young are especially at risk to scalding accidents; the 'reach and pull' type being particularly common. Poorly designed kitchens and unemployed parents may be predisposing factors (Cason, 1990). There is some evidence that at least some ethnic minorities may be at a greater risk of scalding, probably for cultural reasons (Vipulendran et al, 1989).

Table 3. Prime causes of scalds to children admitted to the West Midlands Regional Burns Unit from 1 January 1980 to 30 December 1989.

Age	<5			5–14			All children		
	M	F	P	M	F	P	M	F	P
Baths, buckets etc.	133	109	242	16	23	39	149	132	281
Kettles	144	104	248	20	16	36	164	120	264
Other water spilt	95	59	154	21	20	41	116	79	195
Tea pots	103	59	162	18	6	24	121	65	186
Tea cups	100	76	176	3	8	11	103	84	187
Other hot liquids	106	49	155	6	11	17	112	66	178
Other and unknown	11	9	20	3	3	6	14	12	26
All scalds	692	465	1157	87	87	174	779	552	1331

MINOR BURNS AND SCALDS

Data from the Home Accident Surveillance System suggests that over 100 000 burns and scalds (excluding industrial accidents) occur annually but no distinction is drawn between admitted and outpatient cases. On the basis of two small surveys made two decades ago (Auchincloss, 1975; Lawrence and Bull, 1976) the number of minor burns may be about 10 times those recorded for admitted patients (Lawrence, 1996a). The pattern of causes of minor burns differs from those meriting hospital admission in respect of house fires, flammable liquids and kettle scalds.

SUSCEPTIBILITY TO BURNING

It is commonly said that young children's skin is more susceptible to burns compared with adults but supportive evidence is lacking. However, young children are more susceptible to burning accidents. It is also not widely appreciated that comparatively low temperatures can cause burns (Lawrence and Bull, 1976). The relationship between time and temperature has been explored (Moritz and Henriques, 1947; Lawrence and Bull, 1976) and *Medical Information on Human Reaction to Skin Contact with Hot Surfaces* (BSI, 1983), is available.

BACTERIOLOGY AND INFECTION CONTROL

The microbiology and infection control of burns in children differs little from that of any other population group. These problems have been reviewed (Ayliffe and Lawrence, 1985; Lawrence, 1987b; Sohal, 1996) and useful general infection control information is also available (Ayliffe et al, 1992). By nature, burns readily acquire a range of bacterial species but, over the last 50 years, there has been a decline in the incidence of potentially pathogenic bacteria, which is probably attributable to improvements in infection control generally and topical anti-bacterial prophylaxis in particular (Lawrence, 1992). Earlier reviews (Lowbury, 1978, 1979) of the bacterial problems of burns contain much useful information. Curiously, anaerobic bacteria rarely cause problems in burns (Cason, 1981) although they are not uncommonly isolated from the wound (Lawrence, 1985). Fungi, especially *Candida* spp., are also not uncommon in the wound (Kidson and Lowbury, 1979) yet, in contrast to American experience (Pruitt, 1984), rarely cause clinical problems in the UK (Cason, 1981).

ANTI-BACTERIAL PROPHYLAXIS

Commonly used effective topical prophylactic agents are silver sulpha-diazine cream in conjunction with suitable absorbent dressings or aqueous silver nitrate or povidone iodine for sites that are awkward to dress; few satisfactory proprietary alternatives are available. It is to be remembered that most topical anti-bacterial agents suffer disadvantages (Lawrence, 1985, 1987b). Tulle gras preparations provide an alternative especially for shallow areas, skin graft donor and recipient sites. Medicated versions may be preferable but those containing antibiotics should be avoided. The nature of current tulle gras dressings has been reviewed (Lawrence, 1993).

Antibiotic prophylaxis of burns, apart from by reason of tetanus prophylaxis (which is mandatory), is unnecessary and appears to confer little benefit (Lawrence, 1995; Lawrence and Groves, 1983). For tetanus prophylaxis penicillin is a suitable choice and has the additional benefit of eliminating *Streptococcus pyogenes* should it be present in the patient's throat. *Strep. pyogenes* of Lancefield Group A is particularly pathogenic in burns hence monitoring sore throats of patients, their visitors and staff is desirable. If this organism is isolated from wounds then flucloxacillin is the first choice because a substantial number of burns become colonized with *Staphylococcus aureus*. Erythromycin affords an alternative for penicillin-sensitive persons but its widespread use on a burns unit can result in the emergence of resistant staphylococci (Lilly et al, 1979).

INFECTION

Infection in burns is usually silent (Cason, 1990) but septicaemic episodes can occur at any time during treatment. The classical signs of infection are relatively unusual in burns during the earlier stages of treatment but cellulitis can often be discerned in chronic unhealed areas. The criteria for suspected septicaemia include a temperature exceeding 39.5°C, a lowered blood pressure and an enhanced pulse rate. It should be suspected if the patient is disorientated or the urinary sodium–potassium ion ratio is reversed. Antibiotic therapy should be initiated promptly and not await blood culture results. Although blood cultures are pertinent they are frequently negative, thus therapy usually has to be guided by the wound flora. Since this is usually mixed, broad spectrum antibiotics frequently have to be employed; results can be disappointing. It is to be noted that some patients are likely to be admitted with respiratory problems, often relatively minor, of viral origin and these could account for some of the pyrexic episodes encountered early after burning that can rarely be attributed to any bacterial complication.

The most commonly isolated organisms from blood cultures are *Staph. aureus* and *Pseudomonas aeruginosa* but Gram-negative bacilli such as *Acinetobacter* spp. are also common. Frequently strains of *Staph. aureus* isolated from the burn wound are relatively avirulent but virulent strains can emerge on occasion and become endemic (Lilly et al, 1979). Other staphylococcal problems can occasionally arise such as scalded skin syndrome (Dowsett, 1984), which carries an appreciable mortality (Frame et al, 1985).

Septicaemia is a serious complication of burns such that bacterial infection is a major contribution to burns mortality (Pruitt, 1984). Removal and microscopical examination of biopsies together with quantitative bacteriology is advocated by some (Neal et al, 1981; Pruitt, 1984) to determine evidence of invasive infection—supposedly indicated by bacterial counts exceeding 105 colony forming units/g tissue. The risks associated with this surgical intervention are unknown and the value of biopsies in burn care has recently been questioned by some authorities (Lawrence, 1987b; Steer et al, 1996a,b). Quantitative bacteriological techniques in relation to burns have been reviewed by Sohal (1996).

INFECTION CONTROL

Thorough bacteriological monitoring of burns is desirable but rarely available nowadays especially as microbiological laboratories are often remote from the treatment unit. Hence a good liaison with the laboratory is essential. Schemes for burns bacteriology have been described (Lawrence, 1985, 1987b) but many of the bacteriological problems are not peculiar to burns hence standard microbiological texts (Sleigh and Timbury, 1986; Volk et al, 1996) are also helpful. The potential for cross infection in burns is enormous, consequently thorough attention to all aspects of asepsis and infection control are mandatory. All staff need to be aware of this and trained accordingly. Each unit should produce its own guidance on infection control and use of antibiotics to take account of their own particular problems and to regularly review and update this as circumstances change.

DRESSINGS

Despite the introduction of many innovative dressings in recent years few are suited to the large areas so often encountered in burn care (Lawrence, 1987c). Consequently traditional absorbent cellulose dressings remain the mainstay. A major disadvantage is that such materials are only bacteria proof when dry and this property is lost once they become slightly moist. The use of anti-bacterial creams for topical prophylaxis somewhat extends their useful life. Criteria for changing dressings include: slippage, leakage, strikethrough of exudate, foul smell, swelling of peripheral tissues and unexplained pyrexia. Some authorities also recommend a maximum of 4 days duration (Jeffcott, 1986) but others consider there is no need to change dressings unless any of the problems mentioned occur (Gamgee, 1876; Colebrook, 1950)

Dressings for burns have been reviewed (Lawrence, 1996b) as have dressings in general (Lawrence, 1982, 1990b; Thomas, 1990). Some of the newer dressings are suitable for small burned areas and offer the advantage of being water and bacteria proof (Lawrence, 1990b). It is to be remembered that dressing burns liberates numerous bacteria into the air hence it is recommended practice to use plenum ventilated dressing rooms for this purpose. Even small (1% body surface area) wounds, if colonized, also tend to appreciably increase airborne bacterial numbers. Certain modern dressings can minimize this problem (Lawrence, 1994).

FIRST AID

The first person at the scene of the accident is usually the parent or carer at the time. The treatment that they give to the burnt child can have a considerable effect on the outcome. There is a continuing need for the professionals to ensure that those people caring for children are aware of how to deal with a burn or scald.

Education programmes in the community involving burn care nurses going into schools and involving the children, parents and teachers, have proven to be successful in reducing the number of accidents and improving the initial care. Burned skin cools slowly (Lawrence and Bull, 1976), prompt application of cold tap water rapidly quenches residual heat (Lawrence, 1990a) to minimize damage and reduce pain (Davies, 1982). Most authoritative first aid books and the British Burn Association endorse this advice (Lawrence, 1987a) and the rationale has been discussed (Byrne et al, 1990). Nevertheless, a substantial proportion of admitted cases are not accorded adequate first aid (Petch and Cason, 1993). The cooling process can include cold water, cooling gels or even a packet of frozen peas. It should continue for approximately 10–15 minutes and must be initiated within 20 minutes of the injury to be efficient (Buck et al, 1978).

The depth of a burn is dependent upon the length of time the heat is in contact with the skin (Moritz and Henriques, 1947); by cooling one can limit the total amount of tissue damage. Once the area has been cooled it should be covered by ordinary domestic cling-film. This provides a sterile covering that prevents evaporation from the burn surface, prevents contamination and reduces pain by covering exposed nerve endings.

THE MANAGEMENT OF THE BURN INJURED CHILD IN THE ACCIDENT AND EMERGENCY DEPARTMENT

The main rôle of the Accident and Emergency Department is to assess the child and the injury, initiate treatment, and ensure that the child is safely and promptly transported to a specialist Burn Unit if that is necessary.

ASSESSMENT OF THE AIRWAY

This is especially important if fire has caused the injury. Examination of the nose and mouth can indicate potential airway problems. If the nasal vibrissae are singed and the pharyngeal mucosa is red and injected there has obviously been heat inhalation. Hoarseness of the voice is an indication of damage to the vocal cords.

A history of smoke inhalation can be elicited from the fire brigade. Oedema of the face and neck increases during the first 48 hours and can actually compromise the airway. If there is an immediate need or a strong possibility of there being a need within a few hours then an endotracheal tube should be passed to make the airway safe.

ASSESSMENT FOR THE NEED FOR ANALGESIA

An opioid titrated intravenously is usually the most appropriate analgesia for a moderate to severe injury.

ASSESSMENT OF THE EXTENT OF THE INJURY

This is usually expressed as a percentage of the body surface area and calculated using Lund and Browder charts adjusted to the child's age or simply, if more sophisticated means are not available, by using the patient's hand as representing 1% body surface area. Laser Doppler imaging is an accurate method of assessing size and depth of a burn. Until recently this has been a research tool but is now being used routinely in Burns Units (Niazi et al, 1993). Areas of simple erythema are discounted when calculating the percentage injury. The depth of the injury should be assessed accurately in a small area burn but in a large area it is probably more important to transport the patient to the Burn Unit than spend time in detailed assessment of all the areas. An accurate diagnosis of depth can wait until arrival on the definitive Burn Unit.

All patients must be fully examined to exclude other forms of trauma.

ESTABLISHMENT OF VENOUS ACCESS

Children with burns or scalds involving over 8% of body surface require the insertion of a venous cannula, preferably in a non-injury site. If the patient has poor venous access, then intraosseous fluids should be considered. In an injury involving greater than 10% body surface area, resuscitation should be started using the formula that is appropriate to the Burn Unit involved. In the UK this would usually be a variation of the Muir and Barclay formula using human albumin, for example:

$$\frac{\text{weight in kg} \times \% \text{ body surface}}{2} = \text{ml of colloid solution per period}$$

The resuscitation period extends over 36 hours. In the first 24 hours there are 3×4 hour periods plus 2×6 hour periods. In the second 24 hours there is a 1×12 hour period.

Tetanus prophylaxis should be administered if the child's cover is not up to date.

Very small superficial scalds of an uncontentious nature can be treated in Accident and Emergency Departments. All other patients should be referred to a Paediatric Burn Unit. Small superficial scalds or burns can be dressed with a non-adherent dressing such as chlorhexidine-impregnated tulle covered by an absorbent layer of gauze and bandaged in place. This dressing may be left for 7 days, by which time such a burn will have healed. Children with injuries requiring admission to a Burn Unit should have their wounds covered with cling-film so that the burns can be inspected by the receiving doctor without having to remove dressings and thereby avoiding unnecessary pain and contamination of the burn wound. Patients who are going to have to travel considerable distances to a Paediatric Burn Unit and who have a greater than 10% body surface area injury requiring a resuscitation regimen should be catheterized prior to transportation, as should those patients with burns or scalds involving the vulva or penile skin as swelling can progress rapidly. If the distances involved are small, then the invasive measures may be best left until arrival on the Burn Unit. The child must be kept warm and well perfused.

ASSESSMENT OF POSSIBLE NON-ACCIDENTAL INJURY

This is obviously very important but must be kept in perspective. The needs and safety of the injured child are paramount but the long-term effect of imprudent accusation or investigation should not be forgotten. Within the Accident and Emergency Department the assessment of the family situation can be difficult and is not always appropriate. It is often better left to the admitting Paediatrician. The most important indicator of suspicion of non-accidental injury is when the history or explanation given for the injury does not fit the picture that is being seen on the child. If there is any cause for concern regarding the nature of the injury, there should be a very low threshold for admission to hospital.

BURNS OR SCALDS IN CHILDREN REQUIRING ASSESSMENT IN A BURN UNIT

All injuries in babies under six months.
Superficial scalds over 5%.
All deep dermal injuries.
All full thickness injuries.
Scalds or burns involving the face and neck.
Scalds or burns involving the hands.
All electrical burns.
All chemical burns.
Possible non-accidental injuries, even if of a minor nature.

ROLE OF THE PAEDIATRIC BURN UNIT

The Paediatric Burn Unit gives to the child the advantages of the expertise of burn care professionals in the form of nurse specialists, physio- and occupational therapists, surgeons and anaesthetists, who understand the often very complicated local and systemic disturbances that characterize a burn. These disturbances include fluid and protein loss, wound and systemic infection, gross metabolic, endocrine, haematological and immune disturbance. An understanding of the pathophysiology of the burn wound, wound healing and the achievement of the best long-term results are essential to the management of the burn patient.

RESUSCITATION

All paediatric burn or scald victims with an injury involving over 10% body surface area will become 'shocked' if adequate intravenous resuscitation is not carried out. Unlike other traumatic situations in which shock or loss of fluid is treated by replacement once it has occurred, the key to good burn management is to be ahead of the situation and provide fluid as the fluid loss is occurring. The fluid requirement per percentage burn can be calculated using the Muir and Barclay formula if colloid solutions are preferred (Muir and Barclay, 1962). There are several other formulas available, e.g. Parkhouse. The effectiveness of the resuscitation has to be monitored regularly, usually at the end of each period, using such parameters as haematocrit, full blood count, urea and electrolytes, hourly urinary output, urinary electrolytes and urinary osmolality. The volume of fluid required for the next period is calculated according to the results and, if necessary, calculating the plasma deficit. The formulae therefore should not be considered absolute but used as a guide to patient requirements. Muir has shown that a general relationship exists between the extent of a full thickness burn and the amount of red blood cell destruction. He recommended that when deep burns involve more than 10% of the body surface area, the whole blood requirement is 1% of the patients normal blood volume for each 1% deep burn. It is generally best to give this blood after the first 24 hours.

METABOLIC WATER REQUIREMENT

The amount of salt-free water required by the burn patient is directly related to evaporative and other extra renal losses.

Burns treated by the exposed method lose a considerable amount of fluid by evaporation whereas those treated with dressing lose less fluid. If patients are being nursed on specialist beds, e.g. air fluidized beds, then the extra fluid requirements will have to be taken into consideration.

The water can be given orally if it is well tolerated but otherwise intravenously with 5% glucose solution. The quantity of sodium-free water given should only be sufficient to prevent significant hypernatraemia. If hyponatraemia is allowed to develop intracellular overhydration will occur that can lead on to serious complications. This is the mechanism in many instances of so-called 'burn encephalopathy syndrome' associated with burns and scalds in children. The syndrome includes cerebral irritability, hyperpyrexia, vomiting, twitching, convulsions and coma. It seems that the hyponatraemia results in cerebral oedema and this is one of the factors that produces hypothalamic malfunction so that heat continues to be produced even to the extent of shivering occurring whilst peripheral vaso-constriction continues to minimize heat loss, thus the core temperature rises whilst the shell temperature remains subnormal. If hyperpyrexia occurs it will not respond to external cooling. Treatment should produce peripheral vasodilatation.

THE BURN WOUND

The local effect of a burn is that of tissue damage and destruction. The extent of this damage depends on the temperature and the length of time that this heat has been effective. Clinically the depth of injury is described as:

1. Superficial partial thickness when the hair follicles, sebaceous and sweat glands and the reticular dermis are undamaged. These areas will heal within 7–10 days provided they do not become infected. They are therefore treated conservatively with non-adherent dressings.
2. Deep partial thickness describes an injury when only the deep part of the hair follicles remain intact and the reticular dermis is damaged. Such burns will take longer than 2 weeks to heal.
3. Full thickness burns. These are burns in which all the structures of the skin are damaged by heat.

Clinical assessment of the depth of a burn depends upon the appearance, the presence of capillary return (present in all superficial scalds), the presence or absence of sensation (present in superficial, variable in deep partial thickness and absent in full thickness).

Circumferential full thickness burns require escharotomies as an urgent procedure. This should be done by an experienced surgeon.

The assessment of the depth of the burn can be difficult, even for experienced personnel. The picture is often more definite after 48 hours and so the routine is to reassess the burn wound 2 days after injury.

Objective means of assessing burn wound depth have until recently not been either satisfactory or easily available. Laser Doppler imaging is proving to be a successful tool in the assessment of burn depth and area.

BURN WOUND HEALING

The depth of a burn determines the way in which it will heal. A superficial partial skin thickness injury will heal mainly by re-epithelialization from the remaining epidermal elements, with little contraction. A deep partial skin thickness burn will heal by a mixture of granulation, wound contraction and epithelialization from epidermal remnants and the wound edge. A full thickness burn left to heal will granulate and contract with epithelialization occurring only from the wound edge. This process will take many weeks or months. There is little controversy regarding the superficial wounds that will heal spontaneously, leaving little scarring, providing they are kept clean and in a moist environment. Similarly, no-one would contest that full thickness injuries require debridement and skin graft cover to minimize morbidity and mortality. Deep partial thickness burns can be left to heal spontaneously or can be surgically debrided and skin grafted. Wounds that take longer than 3 weeks to heal have a greater incidence of hypertrophic scarring (Deitch et al, 1983). Wounds that are skin grafted after 14 days also have an increased incidence of hypertrophy within the scar (McDonald and Deitch, 1987). It is therefore reasonable to suggest that deep partial thickness burns that have not healed by 2 weeks should be debrided and skin grafted.

Cytokines TGF-β, EGF, PDGF and IGF-1, have all been shown to accelerate wound epithelialization alone or in combination in animal models (Hunt, 1990). EGF has been shown to do the same in human split skin graft donor sites (Brown et al, 1989) and also to stimulate the healing of chronic wounds, including burn wounds (Brown et al, 1991). For a clinical algorithm of burn wound healing see Figure 1.

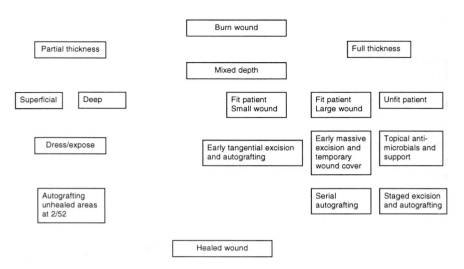

Figure 1. A clinical algorithm of burn wound healing. Reproduced by permission of P. Dzeiwulski.

TREATMENT OF THE BURN WOUND

In clinical practice the burn wound can be treated by conservative methods, surgical intervention, or a combination of both. Conservative management usually consists of the application of dressings usually with topical anti-microbial agents or the wound can by left exposed (in such a situation the patients need to be isolated, which can lead to psychological problems, especially in children). This method of treatment continues until the wound heals, in the case of superficial partial thickness skin burns or in deeper burns until spontaneous separation of the eschar reveals a granulating wound that can be autografted (late surgery).

Surgical management involves the debridement of the non-viable tissue and covering the wound with either skin graft or, in certain cases, if there are exposed nerves, tendons or bone, with a skin flap (Frame et al, 1990). The surgery is usually best carried out early, that is within the first 5 days, or very early, within 24 hours if the wound is very large. The rationale for early aggressive surgery is improved survival and reduced morbidity due to reduced sepsis, hypermetabolism, fluid loss, less pain and hypertrophic scarring (Dziewulski, 1992).

DRESSINGS AND SKIN SUBSTITUTES

The perfect burn dressing would be non-adherent, resist bacterial contamination, be superabsorbent, provide a good environment for wound healing and be of reasonable cost.

Traditionally these dressings have consisted of tulle gras (non-adherent), dressing gauze (absorbent), wool and bandage (barrier to infection). Often anti-microbials are applied to the tulle gras e.g. chlorhexidine or silver sulphadiazine cream.

More recently there has been an influx of synthetic dressings that often produce a better environment for wound healing. One of the disadvantages of these dressings is often the inadequate size to cover a major burn. They can be used on the burn wound during the spontaneous healing phase or on the debrided surface following surgical excision. Biological dressings, consisting mainly of allografts or xenografts are the best dressing for the debrided wound if the patient's own skin is not available. These temporary dressings reduce evaporative water and heat loss from the open wound, thereby preventing desiccation. They also protect the underlying granulating surface and reduce the number of bacteria on the wound surface.

Allograft skin can be obtained from live donors or cadavers after processing, it can be used fresh or stored by different methods, e.g. frozen in liquid nitrogen (Bondoc and Burke, 1971), stored in glycerol (Hermans, 1989) or it can be lyophalized. Availability of allograft skin has recently improved with the setting up of skin banks whose remit is to collect and process the skin and to ensure that it has been screened for communicable diseases, especially those transmitted by viruses (Clarke, 1987).

Xenografts most often in the form of lyophalized pig skin have been available for some time and been extensively used in the management of partial and full thickness burns (Healy and Boorman, 1989). The development of temporary artificial skin substitutes could have great impact on the quality of long-term wound healing in major burns when there is very little in the way of donor skin available.

One such composite biosynthetic substitute has been developed by Burke et al (1981). It consists of silicone elastomeric epidermis and a porous collagen-chondroitin 6-sulphate fibrillar dermis. The dermal portion becomes adherent to the wound and after peeling off the epidermal layer at a later stage it can be covered either with autograft or cultured keratinocytes. The use of this material is very costly but has shown encouraging results (Heimbach et al, 1988).

Cultured keratinocytes in the form of very thin sheets can now be used but in this form do not produce a stable durable skin surface (Woodley et al, 1988). Another disadvantage is the length of time it takes to culture the patients own skin and the problem of how to deal with a major burn wound in the meantime. Research continues in the provision of an artificial dermis onto which the cultured keratinocytes can be placed to improve the durability.

PREVENTION OF WOUND SEPSIS

The burn wound provides an excellent environment for bacterial colonization that can progress to infection and eventually invasive wound sepsis. Invasive sepsis can deepen the effect of the initial injury, progressing a deep partial thickness burn to a full thickness injury. It can also lead to systemic sepsis. The main method of prevention of wound infection is by the application of topical anti-microbials. This has been proven to be more effective than systemic antibiotics. Thus 1% silver sulphadiazine cream is most commonly used on burn wounds. The silver reacts with the DNA of the bacteria and the sulphadiazine has its own bacteriostatic properties. It has some inherent wound healing properties (Penneys, 1982) but has also been shown to be toxic to human fibroblasts (McCauley et al, 1990). Silver sulphadiazine cream changes the appearance of the surface of the burn wound, producing a white slough that makes it difficult to accurately judge the depth. It should therefore not be used until the depth of injury has been ascertained and a decision made as to the need for surgical intervention. The use of cerium nitrate in combination with silver sulphadiazine produces a strongly adherent yellow/green leather-like eschar that preserves dermis in deep partial thickness burns. This persists for many weeks, thereby allowing planned, staged excision of the eschar in large burns, permitting regrowth of donor sites between the operative procedures (Boeckx et al, 1985).

TOXIC SHOCK SYNDROME

Burn children are probably immuno-compromised by their injury and are therefore more likely to be susceptible to the effects of circulating toxins produced by bacterial colonization of their burns (Frame et al, 1987). Staphylococci can produce eight enterotoxins; A, B, C1, C2, C3, D, E and F. Entero-toxin F is also known as toxic shock syndrome (TSS) toxin-1. There need not be active infection in the burn wound for TSS to occur (Holt et al 1987). Toxic shock syndrome can occur in comparatively minor burns and scalds. Clinical early diagnosis and treatment, including aggressive monitoring, intravenous fluids and parenteral anti-staphylococcal therapy are of prime importance (Cole and Shakespeare, 1990). Diagnosis can be based on the following criteria (Cole and Shakespeare, 1990). Pyrexia greater than or equal to 39°C, rash, shock, diarrhoea and/or vomiting, irritability and lymphopenia.

NUTRITION

Burn injury increases the metabolic rate in proportion to the extent and severity of the burn. This increase appears to be mainly due to abnormally high production of catacholamines. It is important to try and reduce the factors that contribute to this hypermetabolic state. It is essential therefore to minimize pain, discomfort and emotional stress and to provide a quiet and restful environment. Heat loss should be prevented by nursing the patient in a warm environment (30–32°C) and to avoid cooling during surgery and dressing changes. Even then a residual hypermetabolism remains that obligatorily requires the production of energy from whatever source is available and continues until the burns are largely healed. Unless adequate nutrition is provided, a considerable negative nitrogen balance is produced and there is a fall in weight due to loss of muscle mass. The calorie and protein intake should be provided by the enteral route if at all possible, thus reducing the translocation of gut flora and the risk of septicaemia from this source. The use of parenteral nutrition runs grave risks of septicaemia.

LONG-TERM EFFECTS OF BURN INJURY

Care of the burned child and their family does not stop once the child has healed and been discharged from inpatient treatment. Experience tells us that children tend to produce hypertrophic scarring despite aggressive early excision and grafting policies. This hypertrophic scarring is combated by means of the application of pressure garments and/or silicone gel sheeting. If these measures are unsuccessful, an injection of Triamcinalone directly into the scar should be considered. This is obviously not feasible in large areas because of dosage restrictions.

Skin contractures are no longer a common problem but when they do occur require release and insertion of either skin grafts or flaps to maintain normal function of the area and normal growth.

Major burn injury can cause psychological stress both to the child and to the family. A Clinical Psychologist is therefore an important member of the burn care team.

The aims of paediatric burn care are to achieve a well-healed, durable, cosmetically acceptable burn wound on a healthy child who is part of a well adjusted family. This outcome is best achieved by the interaction of all the professionals involved in burn care.

REFERENCES

Auchincloss J (1975) Incidence of minor burns. *British Journal of Clinical Practice* **29**: 251–255.

Ayliffe G & Lawrence JC (eds) (1985) Symposium on infection control in burns. *Journal of Hospital Infection* **6 (supplement B)**.

Ayliffe G Lowbury E, Geddes A et al (1992) *Control of Hospital Infection*, (3rd edn) London: Chapman and Hall.

Barrett A (1996) Prognosis. In Settle. J (ed.) *Principles and Practice of Burns Management* pp. 29–42. London: Churchill Livingstone.

Boeckx W, Focquet H, Cornelissen M et al (1985) Bacteriological effect of cerium-flammazine cream in major burns. *Burns* **11**: 337.

Bondoc C & Burke J (1971) Clinical experience with viable frozen human skin and a frozen skin bank. *Annals of Surgery* **174**: 371.

Brown G Nanney L & Griffin J. (1989) Enhancement of wound healing by topical treatment with epidermal growth factor. *New England Journal of Medicine* **32**: 76.

Brown GL, Curtsinger L, Jurkiewicz MJ et al (1991) Stimulation of healing of chronic wounds by epidermal growth factor. *Plastic and Reconstructive Surgery* **88**: 189.

BSI (British Standards Institution) (1983) *Medical Information on Human Reaction to Skin Contact With Hot Surfaces (PD6504)*. London: British Standards Institution.

Buck D, Davis T, Miller S et al (1978) Effect of immediate cooling on tissue extension and volume in the rat (limb) model. *Clinical Research* **26**: A598.

Bull J (1971) Revised analysis of mortality due to burns. *Lancet* **ii**: 1133–1134.

Burke J, Yamas I, & Quinby W et al (1981) Successful use of a physiologically acceptable artificial skin in the treatment of extensive burn injury. *Annals of Surgery* **194**: 413.

Byrne I, Sutcliffe A & Lawrence J (1990) A 'simple and cost-effective' guide to the treatment of burned victims. *Fire* **83**: 19.

Cason C (1990) A study of scalds in Birmingham. *Journal of the Royal Society of Medicine* **83**: 690–692.

Cason J (1981) *Treatment of Burns*. London: Chapman & Hall.

Clarke J (1987) HIV transmission and skin grafts. *Lancet*, **i**: 983.

Cole R & Shakespeare P (1990) Toxic shock syndrome in scalded children. *Burns* **16**: 221–224.

Colebrook L (1950) *A New Approach to the Treatment of Burns and Scalds*. London: Fine Technical Publications.

Davies J (1982) Prompt cooling of burned areas: a review of the benefits and the effector mechanisms. *Burns* **9**: 1–6.

Deitch E, Whelan T, Rose M et al (1983) Hypertrophic burn scars: analysis of variables. *Journal of Trauma* **23**: 895.

Dowsett E (1984) The staphylococcal scalded skin syndrome. *Journal of Hospital Infection* **5**: 347–354.

Dziewulski P (1992) Burn wound healing. *Burns* **18**: 466–478.

Frame J, Eve M, & Hackett M, et al (1985) The toxic shock syndrome in burned children. *Burns* **11**: 234–241.

Frame J, Bird D, & Eve M et al (1987) IgG sub-class levels in thermally injured children. *Scandinavian Journal of Plastic and Reconstructive Surgery* **21**: 323.

Frame J, Taweepokep, Moieman N et al (1990) Immediate fascial flap reconstruction of joints and use of biobrane in the burned limb. *European Burns Journal* **16**: 381.

Gamgee J (1876) The treatment of wounds. *Lancet* **ii**: 885–887.

Healy C & Boorman J (1989) Comparison E–Z derm and Jelonet dressings for partial thickness skin burns. *Burns* **15**: 52.

Heimbach D, Luterman A, Burke J. (1988) Artificial dermis for major burns. A multicentre randomised trial. *Annals of Surgery* **208**: 313.

Hermans M (1989) Clinical experience with glycerol-preserved donor skin treatment in partial thickness burns. *Burns* **15**: 57.

Holt P, Armstrong A, Norfolk G et al (1987) Toxic shock syndrome due to staphyloccal infection of a ER. *Journal of Clinical Practice* **41**: 582.

Hunt T (1990) Basic principles of wound healing. *Journal of Trauma* **30 (supplement)**: S122.

Jeffcott M (1986) The nursing of the burned patient. In Laurence J (ed.) *Burncare*, pp. 87–92. Hull: Smith & Nephew Ltd and the British Burn Association.

Kidson A & Lowbury E (1979) *Candida* infection of burns. *Burns* **6**: 228–230.

Lawrence J (1982) What materials for dressings? *Burns* **13**: 500–512.

Lawrence J (1985) The bacteriology of burns. *Journal of Hospital Infection* **6 (supplement B)**: S3–S17.

Lawrence J (1987a) British Burn Association recommended First Aid for burns. *Burns* **13**: 153.

Lawrence J (1987b) Infection control in burns. In Judkins K (ed.) *Ballière's Clinical Anaesthesiology* vol. 1, pp. 673–692. London: Baillière Tindall.

Lawrence J (1987c) A century after Gamgee. *Burns* **13**: 77–79.

Lawrence J (1990a) Cold water and 'cling film' recommended for first aid treatment of burns victims. *Fire* **83**: 66–67.

Lawrence J (1990b) Bacterial barrier properties of dressings. *Pharmaceutical Journal* **245**: 695–697.

Lawrence J (1991a,) Burn and Scald injuries (Topic Briefing HS 40). Paper presented at the The Royal Society for the Prevention of Accidents, Birmingham.

Lawrence J (1991b) The mortality of burns. *Fire Safety Journal* **17**: 205–215.

Lawrence J (1992) Burn bacteriology during the last 50 years. *Burns* **18 (supplement 2)**: S23–S29.

Lawrence J (1993) Medicated tulle dressings. *Journal of Wound Care* **2**: 240–243.

Lawrence J (1994) Dressings and wound infection. *American Journal of Surgery* **167(1A)**: S21–S24.

Lawrence J (1995) Some aspects of burns and burns research at Birmingham Accident Hospital 1944–93: AB Wallace Memorial Lecture. *Burns* **21**: 403–413.

Lawrence J (1996a) Burns and scalds: aetiology and prevention. In Settle J (ed.) *Principles and Practice of Burns Management*, pp. 3–28. London: Churchill Livingstone.

Lawrence J (1996b) Dressings for burns. In Settle J (ed.) *Principles and Practice of Burns Management*, pp. 259–269. London: Churchill Livingstone.

Lawrence J & Bull J (1976) Thermal conditions which cause skin burns. *Engineering in Medicine* **5**: 61–63.

Lawrence J & Groves A (1983) Are systemic prophylactic antibiotics necessary for burns? *Annals of the Royal College of Surgeons of England* **65**: 279.

Lawrence J & Gowar J (1993) Nightwear fireguards and legislation. Paper presented at the 2nd European Conference on Advances in Wound Management, London.

Lawrence J & Cason C (1994) Kettle scalds. *Journal of Wound Care* **3**: 289–292.

Lilly H, Lowbury E, Wilkins M et al (1979) Staphylococcal sepsis in a burns unit. *Journal of Hygiene* **83**: 429–325.

Lowbury E (1978) Fact or fashion? The rationale of the exposure method, vaccination and other anti-infective measures. *Burns* **5**: 149–159.

Lowbury E (1979) Wits versus genes: the continuing battle against infection. *Journal of Trauma* **19**: 33–45.

McCauley R, Poole B, Heggers J et al (1990) Differential in vitro toxicity of topical antimicrobial agents to human keratinocytes. *Proceedings of the American Burn Association* **22**: 2.

McDonald S & Deitch E (1987) Hypertrophic skin grafts in burn patients: a prospective analysis of variables. *Journal of Trauma* **27**: 147.

Moritz A & Henriques F (1947) Studies of thermal injury. II. The relative importance of time and surface temperature in the causation of cutaneous burns. *American Journal of Pathology* **23**: 695–720.

Muir I & Barclay T (eds) (1962) Treatment of burn shock. In *Burns and Their Treatment*. London: Lloyd-Luke.

Neal G, Lindholm G, Lee M et al (1981) Burn wound histologic culture—a new technique for predicting burn wound sepsis. *Journal of Burn Care and Rehabilitation* **2**: 35–39.

Niazi Z, Essex T, Papini R et al (1993) New laser doppler scanner, a valuable adjunct in burn depth assessment. *Burns* **19**: 485–489.

OPCS (Office of Population Censuses and Surveys) (1991) *1989 Mortality Statistics: Childhood. England and Wales*. London: HMSO.

OPCS (Office of Population Censuses and Surveys) (1992) *1990 Mortality Statistics: Childhood. England and Wales*. London: HMSO.

OPCS (Office of Population Censuses and Surveys) (1993) *1991 Mortality Statistics: Childhood. England and Wales*. London: HMSO.

OPCS (Office of Population Censuses and Surveys) (1995a) *1993 Mortality Statistics: Childhood. England and Wales*. London: HMSO.

OPCS (Office of Population Censuses and Surveys) (1995b) *Mortality Statistics. Fatal Accidents Occurring During Sports and Leisure Activities*. London: HMSO.

OPCS (Office of Population Censuses and Surveys) (1995c) *?? Mortality Statistics: Childhood. England and Wales*. London: HMSO.

Penney N (1982) Inhibition of arachidonic acid oxidation in vitro by vehicle components. *Acta Dermatologie Venereologie* **62**: 59.

Petch N & Cason C (1993) Examining first aid received by burn and scald patients. *Journal of Wound Care* **2**: 102–105.

Pruitt B (1984) The diagnosis and treatment of infection in the burned patient. *Burns* **11**: 79–81.

Roi L, Flora J, Davis T, et al (1981) A severity grading chart for the burned patient. *Annals of Emergency Medicine* **10**: 161–163.

Sleigh J & Timbury M (1986) *Notes on medical microbiology*, 2nd edn. Edinburgh: Churchill Livingstone.

Sohal A (1996) Infection. In Settle J (ed.) *Principles and Practice of Burns Management*, pp. 407–419. London: Churchill Livingstone.

Steer J, Papini R, Wilson A et al (1996a) Quantitative microbiology in the management of burned patients. I. Correlation between quantitative and qualitative burn wound biopsy culture and surface alginate swab culture. *Burns* **22**: 173–176.

Steer J, Papini R, Wilson A et al (1996b) Quantitative microbiology in the management of burned patients. II. Relationship between bacterial counts obtained by burn wound biopsy culture and surface alginate swab culture with clinical outcome following surgery and change of dressings. *Burns* **22**: 177–181.

Thomas S (1990) *Wound Management and Dressings*. London: The Pharmaceutical Press.

Vipulendran V, Lawrence J & Sunderland R (1989) Ethnic differences in incidence of severe burns to children in Birmingham. *British Medical Journal* **298**: 1493–1494.

Volk W, Gebhardt B, Hammarskjold M et al (1996) *Essentials of Medical Microbiology*, 5th edn. Philadelphia: Lippicott-Raven.

Woodley D, Peterson H, Herzog S et al (1988) Burn wounds resurfaced by cultured epidermal autografts show abnormal constitution of anchoring fibrils. *Journal of the American Medical Association* **259**: 2566.

11

Support of the head injured child in the community

ROB FORSYTH PhD, MRCP, DCH

Senior Lecturer in Paediatric Neurology
Department of Child Health, University of Newcastle upon Tyne, Royal Victoria Infirmary, Newcastle upon Tyne NE1 4LP, UK

The stresses of transition to life at home after initial inpatient hospital rehabilitation for a child and family recovering from a traumatic brain injury (TBI) are readily under-estimated. Families still trying to adjust to this recent, abrupt and total upheaval in their circumstances may greet the thought of resuming round the clock care for their injured child at home with considerable apprehension. Such feelings may turn to frustration and anger as they discover the fragmented nature of community provision for their child.

Key words: head injuries, closed; rehabilitation; early intervention (education); education, special; mainstreaming (education); cognitive therapy.

Children who suffer traumatic brain injury (TBI) frequently make a good physical recovery: 'looking good', and giving parents and teachers apparent grounds for expectations of a smooth return to home and school. Such expectations unfortunately often prove over-optimistic. As the reality of the problems of the TBI child dawns, parents often find themselves faced with a situation for which there appears to be little organized provision: their child's needs span the responsibilities of three agencies (health, education and social services) and multiple professions, none of which appears to be taking an overall co-ordinating role. Although the needs of the head-injured adult on returning to the community are increasingly recognized, even the most recent 1996 UK discussion of best practice (Social Services Inspectorate, 1996), merely comments that children's services have not been evaluated. The discrepancy between problem and provision is even more striking for children than for adults (Middleton, 1989).

Effect of age at injury

Despite the now considerable body of evidence to the contrary, a mistaken optimism persists that outcomes for childhood TBI are in general superior to

Baillière's Clinical Paediatrics —
Vol. 5, No. 3, August 1997
ISBN 0–7020–2319–1
0963–6714/97/030479 + 9 $12.00/00

those for similar injuries in adults: a misconception based on naive concepts of greater 'plasticity' in the immature central nervous system (Webb et al, 1996). Such unrealistic expectations in parents and professionals may cause subsequent events to be perceived as academic or employment 'failure'. Importantly they may also lead to inadequate litigation settlements (Johnson, 1992). TBI damage selectively impacts new learning. Unless the brain is mature at the time of injury, TBI can alter a child's entire subsequent developmental trajectory. Such considerations lead to particular concern for the pre-school child sustaining TBI, a relatively unstudied group (Bryan, 1995). The full effects of TBI may not become apparent for some years, and early absence of problems cannot be taken as evidence that they will not evolve: children with TBI can *grow into* a deficit.

Principles of community rehabilitation for children with TBI

The design and provision of services for TBI children is hampered by the ongoing lack of theoretical or empirical trial-based guidance. Despite a recent proliferation of short-term studies, there remain very few controlled, prospective studies of the long-term sequelae of childhood TBI (Klonoff et al, 1995) and meta-analysis of such studies as exist is hampered by lack of uniformity of study populations and outcome parameters. Consequently this review can only sketch broad principles that will need to be adapted to the specifics of particular situations, until they can be better informed by further experimental data.

Which children?

In the UK 150 000 children under 14 with TBI attend hospital each year (Sharples et al, 1990), although there is no simple relationship between hospital attendance or admission and TBI severity and morbidity. There is ongoing controversy about the consequences, if any, of mild head injury not requiring hospital admission. Are these children's risks of long-term sequelae sufficient to warrant follow-up? Wrightson et al (1995) report subtle but definite effects on reading at 6.5 years in pre-schoolers sustaining such mild TBI. Conversely, a cohort study of 6–15 year olds showed no clinically significant deficits at 1 year (Fay et al, 1993). These data may again reflect an inverse relationship between age at injury and outcome. In practice, the numbers of these children are such that offering prospective follow-up will usually be impracticable, and informal school-based surveillance the only feasible form of long-term support (see below). Preliminary efforts at screening mildly injured children for problems likely to affect school re-entry have been reported (Shurtleff et al, 1995), however these tools require highly trained assessors.

An alternative may be to selectively follow children perceived to be at increased risk of late morbidity for a given injury severity. Various studies have suggested that children with pre-morbid emotional, behavioural or cognitive problems are over-represented in TBI populations (for a review, see Oddy, 1993). It appears that such pre-existing factors also affect long-term outcome. Although cognitive outcome appears predominantly determined by injury severity alone; individual and family behavioural and emotional outcomes (which are arguably more pertinent) are very influenced by pre-morbid measures of family functioning (Donders and Ballard, 1996; Rivara et al, 1996). Although such studies raise the possibility of offering follow-up selectively to such families, I know of no studies evaluating such an approach at present.

A family-centred approach

In the long term, it is the 'higher order' cognitive, affective, social and educational consequences of TBI, rather than the more obvious motor and sensory disturbances, that constitute the principal barriers to the ultimate goal of return to maximum potential independence. These disabilities may worsen subtly with time and may not be correctly attributed to the TBI. TBI children and families are thus at real risk that the usual reactive medical paradigm, of referral only if the *status quo* is perceived as unsatisfactory, will fail to identify and tackle needs. Additionally, children may fall foul of ambiguities over division of professional and financial responsibilities between agencies. The only immediate counter-strategy to these problems is first to educate the family itself to watch for potential TBI sequelae; and second to inform them of the practicalities of 'working the system'. These two areas—long-term expectations for outcome, and the availability of resources after hospital discharge—emerge as the greatest areas of perceived informational deficit for caregivers in both adult and childhood studies (Campbell, 1988; McMordie et al, 1991). The rôle of education and advocacy groups (Headway and the Child Head Injury Trust in the UK; and the Brain Injury Association in the USA) is vital.

There will however often be significant impediments to the family taking a pro-active role in rehabilitation. To a greater or lesser extent a full 'bereavement' process must first be completed. Vulnerable parental relationships may fail under this stress. 'The unique awfulness of acquired brain injury is [that the parents] have a daily reminder of the child they lost' (Hall et al, 1990). The life-stage of the family will clearly be significant: the emotions of the family of a head injured adolescent recently destined for university differ from those of the family of an injured 4 year old. Families are generally desperate to get a clear picture from the outset of the problems their child is facing. This can be facilitated from an early stage by giving the family 'full membership' of the rehabilitation team; although care must be taken to give permission for the family to back out and define limits as they feel necessary (Durgin, 1989). The reaction of siblings to the family's focus on the injured child is often an issue, and facilitating communication within the family is vital.

The transition home

For all the failings of current inpatient rehabilitation, many families find the transition to community-centred provision extremely stressful. The lack of quick answers to trivial anxieties in the middle of the night, the sudden change of pace and intensity of therapeutic involvement, perceptions of lack of specific expertise in TBI rehabilitation in the community and, above all, the sense that they are in some sense now 'on their own' are common causes of anxiety. A sense of confrontation with the realities of a child's impairments may be particularly strong at this stage. and continuity of support from the inpatient rehabilitation team through this transition is essential.

COMPONENTS OF COMMUNITY REHABILITATION AND SUPPORT

The ideal provision would be a TBI-specific service centred around the child and family: seamless, and without evident divides between hospital and community services, or between agencies. By contrast the current provision for TBI children and their families is typically characterized by involvement of separate health, education and social service agencies and their respective professions, organizational barriers between hospital and community services, and attempts to meet the needs of the TBI child through available generic disability services. The following discussion recognizes current divisions of responsibility between professions and agencies.

Psychological, psychosocial and emotional support

It has already been emphasized that many aspects of morbidity will only become evident on neuropsychological, and not neurological, examination. Psychologists' involvement in TBI programmes includes both detailed repeated assessments of cognitive function and therapeutic intervention. Estimation of pre-morbid learning difficulties is essential as recovery in these domains may be less likely; however assessment may be hampered by sparse pre-morbid documentation. TBI rarely affects all functions equally: the pattern of deficits is determined by the mechanism of injury. Specific assessment of attention, memory, executive functioning and processing speed is required: any of these domains may be affected and lead to failure to reach potentials predicted by crude global IQ scores. Frontal lobe dysfunction (dysexecutive syndrome), leading to difficulties in independent planning and organizing ('what do I need to take to school tomorrow?') can have a major impact on prospects for long-term functional independence. Unfortunately such difficulties may be least evident under formal test situations with clear demands and fixed structures (Oddy, 1993).

Typical areas for therapeutic intervention include behavioural and social difficulties. Poor 'higher order' social skills (e.g. in interpreting inter-personal situations) can be a problem following major TBI, and may lead to social withdrawal. A renewed dependency on the family also limits opportunities for new outside relationships. Since almost by definition social reintegration happens after discharge, it is almost always left to the family to achieve. Once evident however, social reintegration problems tend to be persistent without targeted intervention. There has been little comparative evaluation of specific techniques (Giles, 1994).

Psychiatric support

Both anxiety and depression are common in TBI survivors, probably due in part to a primary effect of the injury but also as a reaction to perceived social and educational 'failure'. This can lead to an abrupt collapse in psychological well-being, and the ready availability of experienced and motivated child psychiatry liaison is vital to a rehabilitation programme.

Educational issues

Return to employment has been shown to be a very strong predictor of overall quality of outcome in adult TBI studies (Oddy et al, 1985) at least in part by creating opportunities for social interaction and development. However because of the age-at-injury effects discussed above, an initial return to previous educational levels may not be such a useful indicator in childhood TBI. Return to school may be seen as return to normality, but problems may rapidly become apparent, as even mild impairments of attention, information processing speed or problem solving, compounded by irritability and fatigue, affect performance. Such situations require prompt recognition and management if early disillusion is not to set in (Middleton, 1989). To an extent they can be avoided by the creation of individualized education packages with realistic timetables and shortened school days with scheduled rest periods. Identification of specific perceptual or cognitive deficits can inform curriculum planning and presentation of new material.

As previously emphasized, there is a need for ongoing surveillance of children to watch for problems evolving late after TBI, particularly at times of educational transition, such as the under-appreciated challenge of moving from 'learning to read' to 'reading to learn'. For the large numbers of children with milder injuries in particular, the responsibility for informal surveillance in practice falls to educational services. It is important that the fact of a past TBI be retained in children's educational records: failure to attribute a sequence such as distractibility, academic failure and subsequent conduct disorder to a past TBI is probably common. Case control studies of primary age children in special education for behavioural disorders in the USA demonstrated an odds ratio of 3.3 (95% CI 1.3–8.3) for a pre-school TBI episode sufficient to warrant medical attention (Michaud et al, 1993).

Most teachers' expertise lies in training of specific academic skills (such as arithmetic or reading) in children with essentially intact underlying 'deep processes' of reasoning and judgement. In contrast the TBI child may be able to perform previously learned arithmetical or reading tasks deceptively well, but struggle with new learning because of difficulties at this deep level (Carney and Gerring, 1990). This is an area requiring specialist educational expertise (Begali, 1992). TBI can also affect school life outside the classroom, in the challenges of getting the school bus, getting to the next lesson, or even choosing what to eat in the cafeteria.

The child may lack insight that his or her difficulties have a basis in a past TBI, and it is not uncommon for such children to have experienced years of failure without understanding why. Children may construct alternative 'explanations' for their behaviour and difficulties: the home-work they forgot to bring to school was 'stolen'. Insight is vital as without it they can find the responses of others baffling, leading to loss of social confidence (Jacobs, 1993).

Medical responsibilities

A number of well-defined medical complications of TBI need to be actively sought, delineated and, where possible, ameliorated. Motor dyspraxia may be manifest as co-ordination difficulties in both gross and fine motor domains. Sensory deficits, for example sensorineural deafness or optic atrophy, due to involvement of the nerves in skull fractures, are relatively common in severe TBI. The risk of early post-traumatic seizures (3–9%) is higher in paediatric than adult series, although late risk is lower (McLean et al, 1995). Physicians should be vigilant particularly for the impact both of seizures *and anti-convulsant medications*, on cognitive and educational performance. Endocrine dysfunction manifesting as diabetes insipidus or precocious puberty are relatively rare.

DELIVERY OF SERVICES

It is important that the TBI child is seen as a child first, and as head-injured second. The needs of any child, particularly for the proximity of family and community, are paramount. This will normally lead to a drive to deliver services as locally as possible. For the more severely injured child whose interests may be better served by specialist services the balance is however harder to strike.

Community services

In the UK, most districts do not have specialist dedicated TBI services, and provision is usually co-ordinated through child development/disability teams (Crouchman, 1990, 1991). Provision is usually offered within the educational system and although not explicitly stated, the rôle of encourag-ing re-integration into academic and peer-group social life falls to education. This contrasts with the greater North American emphasis on specialist rehabilitation centres with a medical or paramedical ethos.

School-centred approaches have the advantage of usually being locally based. Educators may have known the child pre-morbidly, will be familiar with local provision and will hopefully have established working relation-ships with other agencies and professions in the area. Attention to housing needs will also be facilitated. As previously mentioned, TBI children may perform misleadingly well in highly structured hospital wards, or psychological assessments. The real world problems that have greatest impact on long-term independence, such as executive difficulties and distractibility, are best evaluated in real world settings such as school.

It is important to appreciate however that the generic childhood disability services available in most communities are in many ways not ideally suited particularly to the more severely injured TBI child. Physical disability services are geared largely to the needs of children with relatively static disabilities often acquired in early life. TBI children can demonstrate many different combinations of deficit that may vary significantly with time, requiring a flexibility of provision that such services may find difficult. TBI children do not fit readily into established educational categories of special need. General special educational resources may also be inappropriate: placement of a severely injured TBI child in a Severe Learning Difficulty (SLD) school on the basis of global IQ-based classifications may be very unhelpful as TBI children may have a relatively intact memory of their pre-morbid abilities. Significant gains in ability can be made at rates much greater than other SLD children (Middleton, 1989).

Specialist rehabiliation facilities

In practice the major limitation of community-based services is the intensity of remedial input that can be offered. For those with greater needs, the availability of specialist, centralized services offering intensive input on a day-attender basis may outweigh disadvantages of separation from a local community. Such facilities for more severely injured children are currently underdeveloped in the UK and consequently, a small number of very damaged children currently remain for prolonged periods in general paediatric wards. Such settings not only promote 'illness behaviour', and dependency but may also be found bewildering by severely injured children. The ideal is individual therapy in quiet environments (particularly in the early rehabilitation phase) as free as possible from a 'medical culture'. Adult studies in the UK have suggested a need for 10 rehabilitation places per 250 000 population (Medical Disability Society, 1988). Children might be expected to comprise 10 or 20% of this population. In making such estimates it should be remembered that provision must be made to permit late 're-admissions' that are of proven benefit even several years after an injury (Hall et all, 1990). An important role of such centres will be to provide regional outreach services, and offer training and advisory resources to district teams.

RECOMMENDATIONS: INTEGRATION

The major deficiency of much current provision is its fragmentation. There remain many structural, procedural and professional obstacles to the creation of a seamless service for the TBI child and family and current UK funding mechanisms act as disincentives to collaboration. Collaboration will require common ownership, commitment and clarity of purpose; and creation of coherent management structures: a long-term goal. An interim solution, even if agencies remain administratively separate, is to shield the family of the TBI child from the fragmentation by giving them a single point of contact and continuity: a resource of information and advocacy. The presence of a single point of contact for the early inpatient rehabilitation phase (at present a senior nurse practitioner) has been greatly appreciated by families in our unit. A similar key-worker approach could be adopted in the community.

The predominant role of education services in providing both a rehabilitative environment for the severely injured child, and in ongoing informal surveillance in the mildly injured child has been emphasized. Unfortunately the relative rarity of severe TBI means that teachers are unlikely to gain much individual experience of the educational consequences of TBI. There is great potential in developing the role of specialist advisers within the educational service to act as resources for teachers.

REFERENCES

*Begali V (1992) *Head Injury in Children and Adolescents: A Resource and Review for School and Allied Professionals.* Brandon, Vt: Clinical Psychology Publishing Company.

Bryan MR (1995) The pre-school child sustains a traumatic brain injury: developmental and learning issues. *Neurorehabilitation* **5**: 323–330.

Campbell CH (1988) Needs of relatives and helpfulness of support groups in severe head injury. *Journal of Rehabilitation Nursing* **13**: 320–325.

Carney J & Gerring J (1990) Return to school following severe closed head injury: a critical phase in pediatric rehabilitation. *Pediatrician* **17**: 222–229.

Crouchman M (1990) Head injury—how community paediatricians can help. *Archives of Disease in Childhood* **65**: 1286–1287.

Crouchman M (1991) Children with head injuries. *British Medical Journal* **301**: 1289–1290.

Donders J & Ballard E (1996) Psychological adjustment characteristics of children before and after moderate to severe traumatic brain injury. *Journal of Head Trauma Rehabilitation* **11**: 67–73.

Durgin CJ (1989) Techniques for families to increase their involvement in the rehabilitation process. *Cognitive Rehabilitation* **7**: 22–25.

*Fay GC, Jaffe KM, Polissar NL et al (1993) Mild pediatric traumatic brain injury: a cohort study. *Archives of Physical Medicine and Rehabilitation* **74**: 895–901.

Giles GM (1994) Why provide community support for persons with brain injury. *American Journal of Occupational Therapy* **48**: 295–296.

Hall DM, Johnson SL & Middleton J (1990) Rehabilitation of head injured children. *Archives of Disease in Childhood* **65**: 553–556.

Jacobs MP (1993) Limited understanding of deficit in children with brain dysfunction. *Neuropsychological Rehabilitation* **3**: 341–365.

*Johnson DA (1992) Head injured children and education: a need for greater delineation and understanding. *British Journal of Educational Psychology* **62**: 404–409.

Klonoff H, Campbell C & Klonoff PS (1995) Outcome of head injuries from childhood to adulthood: a twenty-three year follow-up study. In Broman SH & Michel ME (eds) *Traumatic Head Injury in Children*, pp. 219–234. New York: Oxford University Press.

McLean DE, Kaitz ES, Keenan CJ et al (1995) Medical and surgical complications of pediatric brain injury. *Journal of Head Trauma Rehabilitation* **10**: 1–12.

McMordie WR, Rogers KF & Barker SL (1991) Consumer satisfaction with services provided to head-injured patients and their families. *Brain Injury* **5**: 43–51.

Medical Disability Society (1988). The Management of Traumatic Brain Injury—A Working Party Report of the Medical Disability Society, Development Trust of the Young Disabled.

Michaud LJ, Rivara FP, Jaffe KM et al (1993) Traumatic brain injury as a risk factor for behavioral disorders in children. *Archives of Physical Medicine and Rehabilitation* **74**: 368–375.

*Middleton J (1989) Thinking about head injuries in children. *Journal of Child Psychology and Psychiatry* **30**: 663–670.

*Oddy M (1993) Head-injury during childhood. *Neuropsychological Rehabilitation* **3**: 301–320.

*Oddy M, Coughlan T, Tyerman A et al (1985) Social adjustment after closed head injury: a further follow-up seven years after injury. *Journal of Neurology, Neurosurgery and Psychiatry* **48**: 564–568.

Rivara JB, Jaffe KM, Polissar NL et al (1996) Predictors of family functioning and change 3 years after traumatic brain injury in children. *Archives of Physical Medicine and Rehabilitation* **77**: 754–764.

*Sharples P, Storey A, Aynsley-Green et al (1990) Avoidable factors contributing to death of children with head injury. *British Medical Journal* **300**: 87–91.

Shurtleff HA et al (1995) Screening children and adolescents with mild or moderate traumatic brain injury to assist school re-entry. *Journal of Head Trauma Rehabilitation* **10**: 64–79.

*Social Services Inspectorate (1996) A Hidden Disability. Report of the SSI Traumatic Brain Injury Rehabilitation Project, Social Services Inspectorate, Department of Health.

Webb C et al (1996) Age and recovery from brain injury: clinical opinions and experimental evidence. *Brain Injury* **10**: 303–310.

*Wrightson P, McGinn V & Gronwall D (1995) Mild head injury in pre-school children: evidence that it can be associated with a persisting cognitive defect. *Journal of Neurology, Neurosurgery and Psychiatry* **59**: 375–380.

Index

Note: Page numbers of article titles are in **bold** type.